The Institute of Biology's
Studies in Biology no. 135

Neurons and Synapses

D. G. Jones
B.Sc., M.B.B.S., D.Sc., M.I. Biol.
Department of Anatomy and Human Biology,
University of Western Australia

Edward Arnold

First published 1981
by Edward Arnold (Publishers) Limited
41 Bedford Square, London WC1 3DQ

British Library Cataloguing in Publication Data

Jones, D. G.
    Neurons and synapses. – (The Institute of Biology's
studies in biology, ISSN 0537–9024; no. 135)
    1.   Neurobiology
    I. Title   II. Series
    591.1'88   QP355.2

ISBN 0 7131 2825 9

Photoset and printed by Photobooks (Bristol) Ltd.

General Preface to the Series

Because it is no longer possible for one textbook to cover the whole field of biology while remaining sufficiently up to date, the Institute of Biology proposed this series so that teachers and students can learn about significant developments. The enthusiastic acceptance of 'Studies in Biology' shows that the books are providing authoritative views of biological topics.

The features of the series include the attention given to methods, the selected list of books for further reading and, wherever possible, suggestions for practical work.

Readers' comments will be welcomed by the Education Officer of the Institute.

1981   Institute of Biology
                                              41 Queen's Gate
                                              London SW7 5HU

Preface

Few areas of modern biology are in such ferment as neurobiology, and few areas are as forbidding to the non-specialist as neurobiology. The success of research endeavours in this burgeoning area has tended to make the subdisciplines into which it is divided inaccessible to outsiders. The present book is an attempt to overcome this obstacle by viewing two of the basic components of the nervous system – neurons and synapses – within the perspective of the nervous system as an entity. To accomplish this the topics considered range from the macroscopic to the ultrastructural and encompass morphological and biochemical approaches.

Issues and problems are raised whenever necessary; some currently-accepted interpretations are critically analyzed. Ideas expressed here should not be regarded as final. Many will undoubtedly undergo considerable revision within the coming years. Nevertheless, present concepts are important because they are the only ones we have; they are to be bettered rather than glibly discarded. My hope is that the reader will be prepared to question interpretations as a prelude to constructive thinking.

I am grateful to Mrs Barbara Telfer and Ms Donna Redl for help with the diagrams, to Mrs Susan Dyson for providing the electron micrograph and to TVW Telethon Foundation (Western Australia) for support with aspects of this and other neurobiological projects.

Perth, 1981   D.G.J.

Contents

1 Organization of the Central Nervous System

The focus of this book is the neuron, with particular emphasis on the synaptic connections between neurons. Nevertheless, it would be unwise to limit attention prematurely to these specific components of the nervous system, because to do so would obscure the role of the neurons and synapses in making the nervous system such an immensely complex and refined instrument. Indeed, an understanding of the organization and connectivity of neurons is essential for an understanding of brain function as a whole.

The transition from the level of neurons to that of consciousness and all that is characteristic of human thought, human values and human culture is an immense one. Moreover, it would be grossly misleading to suggest that the bridging of this transition had been accomplished; it has only just commenced. Nevertheless, the neurons and their environment provide a perspective within which many features of brain organization can be usefully approached. In particular, the nature of brain plasticity can be profitably explored against a background of neuronal and synaptic plasticity. Movement between the microscopic and macroscopic levels of organization is essential therefore, if the full potential of the explanatory power of neurons and synapses is to be realized. Hence the need for an initial introduction to the general features of the nervous system in its entirety.

1.1 Overview

Together, the brain and spinal cord constitute the *central nervous system* (CNS), which is kept in contact with the receptors and effectors of the rest of the body by the *peripheral nervous system*. The nerves of the latter convey messages to and from the spinal cord. Afferent nerves run towards the cord and have a sensory function, whereas efferent nerves run away from it and are motor. Afferent nerves carry information about sensations at the surface of the body in to the spinal cord, while efferent nerves bring about the movements of muscle groups, thereby bringing the limbs and trunk into action.

The peripheral nerves are subdivided into two groups: spinal nerves connected to the spinal cord, and cranial nerves connected to the brain.

Spinal nerves are arranged segmentally, one pair to each body segment. Each nerve is connected to the spinal cord by a dorsal and ventral root, and contains both sensory and motor fibres. There are twelve pairs of cranial nerves, all of which originate from the brain and leave the cranial cavity to be distributed to structures principally in the head and neck region. The nerves have sensory and motor components of somatic (bodily), visceral (organs) and special visceral fibres.

A third component of the nervous system is the *autonomic nervous system*, which is concerned with controlling the body's involuntary activities. These include such functions as the beating of the heart, movements of the gastrointestinal tract, and the secretion of sweat. Although these activities have traditionally been regarded as involuntary ones, this may be a misnomer, as biofeedback research indicates that it is possible for individuals to exert some conscious control over them.

The autonomic nervous system is subdivisible into two parts: sympathetic and parasympathetic. The fibres of both systems arise from neurons of the visceral columns of the brain and spinal cord, and synapse with ganglion cells in the periphery before reaching the organs they supply. The respective fibres, however, leave the CNS at different sites, those of the sympathetic system in the thoracic and upper lumbar regions of the spinal cord and those of the parasympathetic system at the cranial (head) and sacral (lower) ends of the CNS. In general, the fibres of the two systems have opposing effects on the organs they innervate, most organs being supplied by both systems. The sympathetic system, for instance, accelerates the heart, constricts arteries, slows gastrointestinal movements and contracts various sphincters. The fibres of the parasympathetic system exert precisely opposite effects.

1.2 Spinal cord

Information entering the spinal cord via afferent (sensory) nerves generally passes to the butterfly-shaped grey matter of the spinal cord (Fig. 1–1). Here the incoming nerve fibre usually synapses with a second fibre, which transports the information upwards within the white matter of the cord to the thalamus. A further synaptic connection occurs in the thalamus, and a final neuron conveys the information to the sensory part of the brain's cerebral cortex. Most ascending tracts, as these are called, cross from one side of the spinal cord to the other somewhere along their course. The major ascending tracts are the anterior and lateral *spinothalamic tracts* (Fig. 1–1), carrying pain, touch and temperature sensations; the *posterior columns*, responsible for conscious position sense, vibration, and size and shape discrimination; and the anterior and posterior *spinocerebellar tracts*, carrying information on unconscious position sense.

Once an appropriate response has been determined within the brain, information is sent back to the spinal cord via another set of tracts. These are the *descending tracts*, which are again found in the white matter of the brainstem and spinal cord. The major one is the corticospinal (pyramidal) tract, responsible for conveying commands for voluntary movement from the motor cortex of the brain (§ 1.3) to the spinal cord (Fig. 1–1). This subdivides into two constituent tracts – lateral and anterior – in the lower part of the brainstem. Most of the corticospinal fibres cross over from one side of the CNS to the other, with the result that the left side of the brain controls movements of the right side of the body, and *vice versa*.

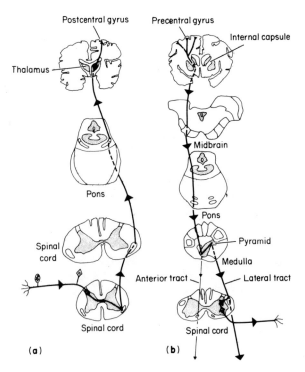

Fig. 1-1 Diagrams illustrating (**a**) lateral spinothalamic tract, and (**b**) corticospinal tract. The lateral spinothalamic tract originates from temperature and pain receptors of the skin, and terminates in the sensory cortex. The corticospinal tract originates from the motor cortex and descends to the spinal cord.

1.3 Brain

The human brain can be subdivided into three principal regions: *forebrain*, *midbrain* and *hindbrain*. The forebrain can be further subdivided into the cerebral hemispheres and the more deeply-situated thalamus, while the hindbrain consists of the pons, medulla and cerebellum (Fig. 1-2).

The cerebral hemispheres are joined together across the midline by a bundle of fibres, the *corpus callosum*. Each hemisphere consists of a core of white matter and a 3–4 mm thick enveloping rind of grey matter, the cerebral cortex. The surface of the hemispheres is characterized by numerous fissures (sulci) between which are folds (gyri). The purpose of this irregularity is to increase the surface area of the hemispheres and hence the area of the cerebral cortex. From the side each cerebral hemisphere displays frontal, occipital, parietal and temporal lobes, separated by sulci (Fig. 1-3). Functionally-distinct regions within the cerebral hemispheres include motor, sensory, visual, auditory and olfactory

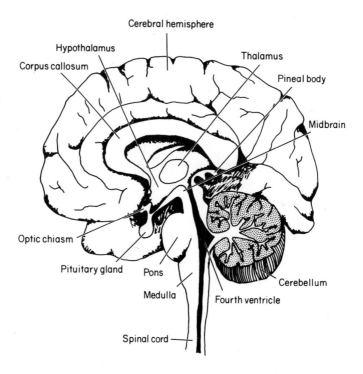

Fig. 1–2 Vertical section of the human brain in the midline, displaying medial views of brain regions.

areas, plus Broca's and Wernicke's speech areas (generally in the left hemisphere).

Deeply embedded within each cerebral hemisphere are the nuclei of the *basal ganglia*, which are intimately involved in the execution of voluntary movements. In the vicinity of the basal ganglia is the *thalamus*; one of the chief functions of this intricate structure is to act as a final relay station where ascending, sensory influences are processed before transmission to the sensory region of the cerebral cortex. It is also implicated, with the cerebellum, basal ganglia and motor cortex, in motor control. The *hypothalamus* lies alongside the thalamus (Fig. 1–2) and plays an important role in the regulation of the autonomic nervous system as well as of various endocrine glands.

The *midbrain* is by far the smallest subdivision of the brain, consisting of various nuclei and fibre tracts. The latter are made up of nerve fibres on their way to the forebrain or hindbrain. The functions served by these structures include control of visual and auditory reflexes.

The *hindbrain* is continuous with the upper end of the spinal cord, and consists of the *pons*, the *medulla oblongata*, and on either side of these the *cerebellum* (Fig.

1-2). Numerous fibres decussate in some part of the hindbrain, running from one side of the brainstem to the other.

Deep within the substance of the brain and spinal cord is a series of cavities, the *ventricular system*, the function of which is to produce cerebrospinal fluid and circulate it within and around the brain and spinal cord. In this way the CNS is bathed in a fluid environment, which to some extent protects it from external injury. The lateral ventricles lie within the cerebral hemispheres, the third ventricle close to the thalamus, and the fourth ventricle within the pons and medulla (Fig. 1-2). These ventricles are connected to one another by small channels, and by foramina, with a subarachnoid space around the brain and spinal cord.

1.4 Cerebral cortex

Microscopical examination of the cerebral cortex demonstrates that neurons are not homogeneously distributed throughout the cerebral cortex. Furthermore, they are of two major varieties, *pyramidal* and *stellate* cells (Fig. 1-4). The pyramidal cells range in size from small ones, 10-12 μm in height, to large ones, up to 100 μm high. The latter giant pyramidal cells are characteristic of the motor cortex. The upper end of the pyramidal cell continues toward the cortical surface as an apical dendrite; this is covered with numerous spines and hence makes numerous synaptic contacts (§ 2.2) The axons of the pyramidal cells pass to other cortical areas, to the opposite hemisphere, or to subcortical, brainstem and spinal cord regions.

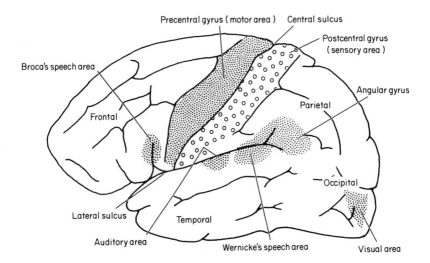

Fig. 1-3 Left cerebral hemisphere of the human brain showing the major lobes into which it is divided, plus the localization of functionally-distinct areas.

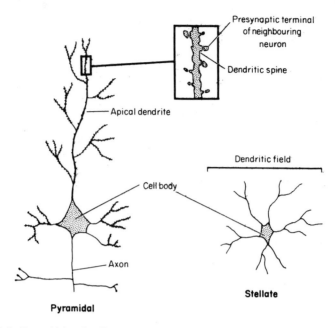

Fig. 1–4   Pyramidal and stellate neurons in Golgi-stained preparations. The inset shows enlarged dendritic spines. The dendritic field refers to the spread of the dendrites of each neuron.

The stellate (granule) cells have oval or circular cell bodies, and a short axon. They lack a major apical dendrite, while their other dendrites make few synaptic contacts. These cells function principally as interneurons, linking up other neurons.

Diversity within the cerebral cortex is accomplished by the manner in which these cell types are distributed throughout the cortex. In most cortical regions six layers can be recognized. The most superficial is the molecular layer, with few cell bodies and a vast array of axodendritic synapses (§ 4.2). The deeper layers differ from each other in terms of their content of variously-sized pyramidal and granule cells. Underlying the deepest layer iş the white matter of the cerebral hemispheres, which consists of nerve fibres running between different regions of the CNS. Of these fibres the *commissural* traverse the midline and connect equivalent centres in the two hemispheres. The largest of these commissures is the corpus callosum, containing 200 million fibres (Fig. 1–2). Cutting these fibres prevents information in one hemisphere from spreading to the other. *Association* fibres are confined to a particular hemisphere, and connect gyri of the same hemisphere. Lesions of them give rise to deficits in memory and speech. *Projection* fibres either arise in the cerebral cortex and end in subcortical regions, brainstem and spinal cord, or run in the opposite direction.

2 Neurons

2.1 Neuron doctrine

One of the greatest obstacles encountered by neurobiologists in their study of the mammalian brain has been its complexity. For morphologists this has entailed the arduous task of wading through entangled networks of neuronal processes, in an attempt to bestow order and pattern on the seemingly disordered. It was the neurohistologists of the latter part of the nineteenth century who did precisely this, as they attempted to decide whether neurons were discrete entities or simply part of an extensive network of fibres and processes. These two possibilities were known, respectively, as the *neuron* and *reticular* theories, and each had its ardent champions. Perhaps the best-known of these were Santiago Ramon y Cajal, the main protagonist of the neuron theory, and Camillo Golgi with his insistence that the neurons constitute an integral part of a continuous network or reticulum.

The anachronism of this controversy lay in the fact that it was Golgi's new staining methods, coupled with Cajal's brilliant concepts, that led to the triumph of the neuron theory. The advent of Golgi's silver staining method in 1873 placed neurohistology on a new footing by providing it with vastly superior preparations. It was left to Cajal and a few others to utilize Golgi's techniques to the full. Between 1888 and 1933 Cajal produced a spate of papers establishing that the functional connections between neurons are brought about by their close contact.

So it was that the era of synaptology was born, although as early as 1897 Sir Charles Sherrington, doyen of English neurophysiologists, had coined the term, *synapse*, in an attempt to explain the characteristic features of the reflex arc. While Sherrington's use of the term had a firm grounding in morphology, he used it in a functional sense to denote those areas of close contact between neurons specialized for effective transmission from the one to the other. Underlying the word itself is the notion of one neuron 'clasping' another or, more specifically, the axon of one clasping the dendrite or cell body (soma) of another.

Light microscopy in the first half of this century stemmed from the development of staining techniques such as the reduced-silver, methylene-blue-vital, Golgi and Nissl methods.

Silver-stained preparations highlight axonal terminations on cell bodies and dendrites. The terminations stand out as synaptic boutons on account of their content of either mitochondria or neurofilaments, depending on the stain used. *Boutons* are characterized as ring-, bulb- and club-shaped profiles (Fig. 2–1);

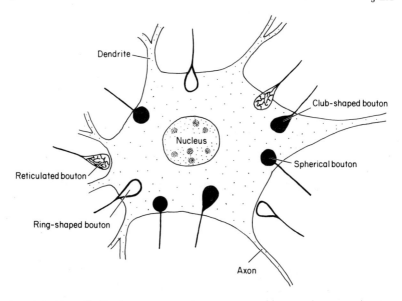

Fig. 2-1 Neurofibrillar boutons on a spinal cord ventral horn cell. Note the different shapes of the boutons, although there is little indication of their substructural organization. This is a diagrammatic representation of a silver-stained preparation, which stains the neurofilamentous bundles in the boutons.

hence the position and number of synaptic contacts can be determined, but little can be said about internal structure.

Of greatest interest in contemporary terms are Golgi preparations, in which some complete neurons, including their cell body and processes, are stained. These were brilliantly exploited by Cajal at the turn of the century, and it was his use of this range of techniques that enabled him to lay the basis of so much CNS circuitry, and opened the way to the classification of neuronal types. At higher magnifications, numerous spines can be recognized over dendritic surfaces (Fig. 1-4), and these mark the sites at which synaptic contacts occur between the dendrites of one neuron and the axons of adjacent ones.

In the 1870s Du Bois-Reymond suggested that neurotransmission may be either chemical or electrical in nature, but it was left to Elliott and later to Dixon in the early 1900s to suggest that a chemical transmitter might be released at the nerve endings, sympathetic nerve impulses liberating adrenaline and parasympathetic impulses a muscarine-like substance.

In 1914 Sir Henry Dale discovered acetylcholine (ACh). He speculated that it may have physiological significance because of its resemblance to the actions resulting from parasympathetic stimulation. At this stage there was no evidence for the liberation of either ACh or adrenaline at the nerve endings, a gap which was partially filled by Otto Loewi when he demonstrated the release of ACh during stimulation of the vagus nerve with subsequent inhibition of the heart. The sympathetic side of the story was provided ten years later by Cannon and Bacq in 1931.

Further work by Dale and others led to the extension of the chemical transmitter hypothesis to sympathetic ganglia and neuromuscular junctions with ACh as the transmitter. In 1935 Dale proposed that the chemical transmitter hypothesis also be applied to synapses of the CNS, an event of great significance for subsequent neurochemical and neuroanatomical studies.

2.2 Neuronal morphology

Neurons show a considerable degree of diversity depending on the number and arrangement of the dendrites. The result is multipolar, bipolar, unipolar and apolar neurons.

Multipolar neurons are the most frequently encountered and are characterized by the possession of a single axon and a number of dendrites. Arrangements vary, and include some cells with a symmetrical spread of dendrites around the cell body, and others with dendrites confined to specific regions above and below the cell body. *Bipolar neurons* have two processes – an axon and a dendrite – arising from the cell body. They are sensory in function, and are found in the retina, nasal passages and receptors of the inner ear. *Unipolar* neurons are characterized by a single process, serving as axon and dendrite; they are far more common in the invertebrate than the vertebrate nervous system, where they occur in sensory ganglia. Neurons lacking any process at all, *apolar neurons*, occur during early development.

Neurons are sometimes distinguished on the basis of axon length. Golgi type I neurons have long axons and Golgi type II short ones (Fig. 1–4). Of these two varieties, the Golgi type II are the more common constituting the internuncial (connecting) cells of the CNS. The long axons of the Golgi type I neurons form the tracts and commissures of the CNS.

In most vertebrate neurons the dendrites conduct impulses towards the cell body, while the axon conducts impulses away from it. The axon often possesses a myelin sheath as insulation, the dendrites never do.

In general, dendrites of adult neurons are fairly short processes with a length of about 1 mm. In multipolar neurons the dendrites branch repeatedly as they move away from the cell body giving to the dendrites a tree-like appearance – the dendritic field (Fig. 1–4). The branching of dendrites is consistent for many types of neuron, so that the number and distribution of first-, second- and third-order dendrites are consistent for a given type of neuron at a particular age. As a result, they provide clues to the state of maturity of the neurons; since these are readily quantifiable features, they are proving of value in experimental studies dealing with, for instance, the effects of malnutrition, sensory deprivation and hypothyroidism on normal brain development.

Dendritic spines consist of a neck and terminal swelling, and constitute the postsynaptic component of axodendritic synapses (§ 4.1). They are generally found on dendritic branches, but are absent from the more proximal part of dendritic trunks. In some neurons they account for almost half the total neuronal surface area, reaching lengths of 1–5 μm and occurring in numbers of 40 000–100 000 per cell. Dendritic spines lack microtubules and neurofilaments, although they frequently contain an enigmatic spine apparatus (§ 4.1).

The axon is the thinnest and longest process of a neuron, the length varying from 200 μm to at least one metre depending on the type of neuron under consideration. The profuse branching of the dendrites does not occur in axons, although a few collateral branches may be present (Fig. 1–4). Most axons arise directly from the cell body, the region of origin being the axon hillock (Fig. 2–2). This, in turn, merges with the initial segment of the axon, which is distinguished from the remainder of the axon by its lack of a myelin sheath. Within the axonal cytoplasm are numerous mitochondria, as well as profiles of smooth endoplasmic reticulum, microtubules and neurofilaments. Situated at intervals along myelin-ensheathed axons are nodes of Ranvier, where the myelin lamellae terminate, leaving an exposed section of axon.

The axon transports proteins and neurotransmitter materials from the cell body toward the terminal. There is movement of the axoplasm itself (axonal flow), of the order of 1 mm per day. Besides this, axonal transport within the axoplasm takes place, representing a much more rapid means of conveying substances along the axon. For instance, some light protein particles travel up to 150 mm per day. Such fast intra-axonal transport is probably brought about by the microtubules, a phenomenon made possible perhaps by a sliding-vesicle mechanism.

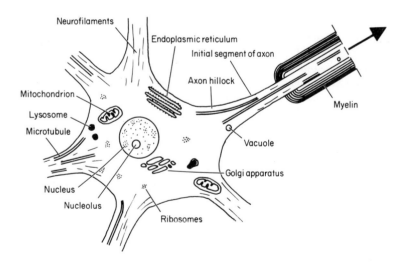

Fig. 2–2   Diagram of a neuron showing its major cytoplasmic constituents, and the component parts of an axon. Arrow indicates direction of nerve impulse.

Within the neuronal cell body is a centrally-located nucleus (Fig. 2–2). Typically, this is large and ovoid, with a single spherical nucleolus that stains strongly for RNA and DNA. The cytoplasm contains organelles that provide the metabolic requirements of the cell. These organelles include Nissl substance, Golgi apparatus, mitochondria and various inclusions. The bulk of the neuronal cytoplasm is produced in the cell body, and from here is distributed to the axon and dendrites.

The Nissl substance is a light microscope phenomenon demonstrated using basophilic stains. With the electron microscope it appears as parallel rows of endoplasmic reticulum plus associated ribosomes (Fig. 2–2). The Nissl substance is most concentrated in the cell body and adjacent parts of dendrites. Besides the ribosomes associated with endoplasmic reticulum, others lie free in the cytoplasm scattered throughout the cell body, dendrites and the initial part of the axon closest to the cell body. Since ribosomes are the principal sites of protein synthesis, much of the protein is produced in the cell body from where it is transported along the axon to its synaptic termination.

The Golgi apparatus is demonstrated at the light microscope level with osmium and silver stains. Ultrastructurally, it appears as a series of stacks of smooth membranes, located in the cell body and proximal regions of dendrites (Fig. 2–2). The protein secretion from the Nissl substance is transferred to the Golgi apparatus, where a carbohydrate component is added before release as secretory vesicles.

Additional structures present in the neuronal cytoplasm include mitochondria, lysosomes, various inclusions, microtubules, neurofilaments and microfilaments. Of these, the mitochondria are responsible for the energy production required for metabolic functions, while the lysosomes have a role to play in the digestion of macromolecules. The inclusions include pigment, glycogen and lipid droplets.

Microtubules are long tubes along the length of the neuron, traversing the dendrites and axon (Fig. 2–2). They are 25 nm in diameter and appear to function as a skeleton for the neuron, thereby maintaining the characteristic shape of the different cell types. In addition, they probably serve a transport role by providing a means by which materials may be transported along the axon and dendrites from the cell body towards their terminations, and also in the opposite direction. Microtubules consist principally of the protein, tubulin, which binds to drugs such as colchicine and vinblastine.

Neurofilaments are of the order of 10 nm in diameter and are distributed throughout the neuron. They occur in some dendritic spines, where they have a ring-like orientation. They also increase in number and may largely fill terminals which are degenerating. The function of neurofilaments is not clear, although it has been suggested they help form the neuronal skeleton.

Microfilaments are slightly smaller than neurofilaments, with a diameter of around 6 nm. They predominate in the developing neuron, and are probably responsible for neuronal movements.

2.3 Neuroglia

A discussion of the architecture of the nervous system is incomplete without reference to the neuroglia or supporting cells, which bind together the neuronal material. However, in spite of the fact that there are as many as 6–10 neuroglial cells for each neuron in the CNS, the neuroglia are easily overlooked. This may, in part, be accounted for by the difficulties sometimes experienced in distinguishing between neurons and neuroglia at the ultrastructural level.

The neuroglia of the CNS can be divided into three types: astrocytes, oligodendrocytes and microglia (Fig. 2–3). Their counterpart in the peripheral nervous system is a single cell type, the Schwann cell. They constitute a dynamic system of functional significance in fluid and respiratory interchange between the neurons and their environment. They form the structural matrix of the CNS

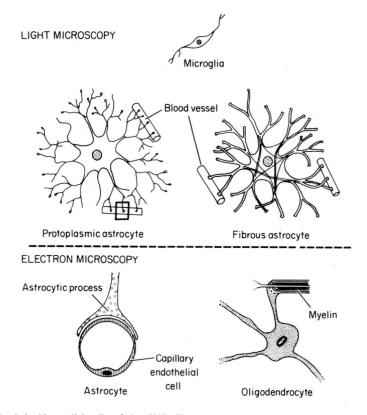

Fig. 2–3 Neuroglial cells of the CNS. The astrocyte processes and capillary at the electron microscope level (lower left) are enlargements of the boxed-in area of the protoplasmic astrocyte (upper left).

and play a vital part in transporting gas, water, electrolytes and metabolites *to* neurons and waste products *away from* them. A major difference between neurons and glia is that, while neurons are generally incapable of undergoing regeneration in the adult CNS, glial cells can be regenerated.

Astrocytes are small, rounded cells with large numbers of radiating processes (Fig. 2–3). They occur in all parts of the CNS, and are subdivided into two types – protoplasmic and fibrous. Of these, the protoplasmic astrocytes have many branching processes and are found predominantly within the grey matter of the brain and spinal cord. The fibrous astrocytes, by contrast, have longer, more slender processes characterized by numerous cytoplasmic fibrils. They occur principally in the white matter.

One of the distinguishing features of astrocytes is the manner in which they intermingle with the processes of neurons, thereby separating neuronal processes from each other. As a result, their shape is derived from their relationship to surrounding neuronal profiles. At the ultrastructural level they have a watery appearance, with few organelles. Some astrocytes surround blood vessels, bestowing upon the vessels a perivascular limiting membrane.

Functionally, astrocytes provide essential nutrients for neurons, form the blood-brain barrier, remove degenerative debris, and insulate unmyelinated neural processes from each other.

The *oligodendrocytes* are the most frequently-encountered variety of neuroglia, and stand out by virtue of their relative lack of cytoplasmic processes; their most prominent feature is a darkly-staining nucleus (Fig. 2–3). They form and maintain myelin, with any one oligodendrocyte providing the myelin sheaths of a number of axons.

Microglia serve as multipotential cells. They can act as phagocytes, removing degenerative material from sites of focal degeneration in the brain.

3 Neural Development

3.1 Organogenesis

The nervous system first appears very early in gestation with the 'heaping up' of ectodermal cells, and the subsequent development of the notochord. The ectoderm overlying the notochord thickens to form the *neural plate*, on either side of which is a strip of ectoderm, the neural crest (Fig. 3–1). The neural plate invaginates to produce the neural groove, which gradually deepens and eventually closes to form the neural tube. The latter is a fluid-filled space, initially open at both ends but ultimately closing off.

Alongside this development, the adjacent neural crest separates from the overlying ectoderm. The neural crest cells appear as an almost continuous column of cells and eventually give rise to the constituent parts of the peripheral nervous system. The CNS is derived from the neural tube.

Further development of the neural tube is effected by repeated cell divisions of the cells in its wall. The result at the macroscopic level is the ballooning out of the rostral (head) end of the neural tube to form three dilatations. These are the

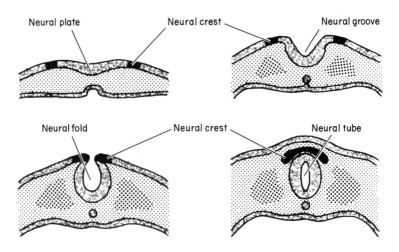

Fig. 3–1 Development of neural tube from neural plate. Neural crest cells are also shown.

major subdivisions of the brain, the *primary vesicles*, representing the forebrain (prosencephalon), midbrain (mesencephalon) and hindbrain (rhombencephalon). The caudal (tail) part of the neural tube develops into the spinal cord.

In subsequent development the prosencephalon becomes further subdivided into the telencephalon (cerebral hemispheres) and diencephalon (mainly thalamus). The mesencephalon remains as a single entity, while the rhombencephalon divides into metencephalon (pons and cerebellum) and myelencephalon (medulla). The cavity of the neural tube develops into the ventricular system.

At the same time as the future regions of the brain are undergoing demarcation, the brain as a whole is bending. The end result is an adult CNS bent at almost right-angles at the mesencephalic-diencephalic junction.

One quite different feature is the development of fissures (sulci) on the surface of the cerebral hemispheres (a typical human characteristic). The first fissures appear at 19 weeks' gestation. By term most of the fissures are present, although both they and the gyri increase in size with further neuronal differentiation.

An important concept in organogenesis is that of the *growth spurt*. The brain grows especially rapidly over a well-defined period of time, either in late foetal or early postnatal life. In the rat it occupies the first three weeks of postnatal life, whereas in the human it is divided into pre- and postnatal components, extending from the end of the second trimester of pregnancy until well into the second year of postnatal life.

Neuronal multiplication takes place prior to the growth spurt, the latter commencing once the full (adult) complement of neurons has largely been attained. The growth spurt itself is characterized by the outgrowth of axons and dendrites and the consequent establishment of synaptic connections, the multiplication and enlargement of glia, and the production of myelin (Fig. 3-2).

Interruption to the growth spurt will affect these three processes but will have little effect upon the number of neurons. Deficits in gross features of the brain, such as brain weight and cortical thickness, will be the result therefore of various factors, principally deficits in the numbers and characteristics of glia, myelin and neuronal connections.

These concepts are based on experimental indices, which include gross parameters such as brain weight, ratio of brain weight to body weight, and thickness of the cerebral cortex, and cellular parameters such as total cell number and cholesterol level (marker of myelin formation). While measurements of indices like these have proved of considerable value for brain growth studies, they have limitations. For example, it is not clear what information these indices convey about the brain as a functioning unit, and individual indices are not generally related to each other in a simple one-to-one manner.

Interest in gross parameters has a much longer history than debate about the growth spurt. *Brain weight*, in particular, has been regarded as a paradigm for the anatomical study of the developing brain, with its typical increase in brain weight. This is especially pronounced in the neonatal period (first eight postnatal days in the rat). While brain weight is readily measured, its usefulness as a parameter of brain development is difficult to determine. It has not proved

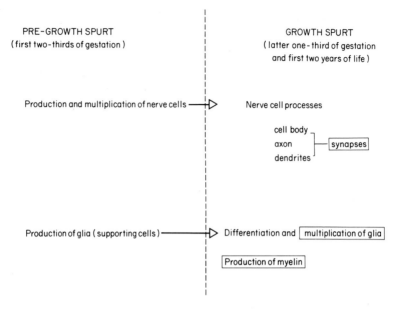

Fig. 3-2   Components of pre-growth spurt and growth spurt. The gestation periods refer to human gestation.

possible to demonstrate a correlation between it and neuronal number. Nevertheless, some correlation may exist between brain weight and body weight.

Cortical thickness is a surprisingly reliable index of brain maturation. In the rat it increases rapidly over the first ten days of postnatal life, with negligible growth thereafter. It can also be roughly correlated with other parameters such as cortical area, cerebral width and even brain width at specific ages during development.

The *water content* of the brain decreases with increasing age, reaching a minimum level at about 50 days in the rat. Accompanying these changes are concomitant ones in the extracellular space, which decreases progressively during maturation. The extent of the decrease depends to some degree on the method used to measure it, although physiological methods, and measurements of the chloride and inulin spaces all record decreases of the order of 20 per cent. Extracellular spaces probably serve as channels for the diffusion of ions and metabolites; they are particularly important in early development as the number of functioning blood vessels is low at that time.

With the development of neuronal processes and the maturation of glia there is a decrease in *cell packing density* during early development. Another useful index is the *glia/neuron index*, which increases rapidly during the growth spurt, partly due to an absolute increase in glial numbers and partly a result of a decrease in the number of neurons per unit volume. Neuron packing density in the rat decreases from 145 000 cells mm^{-3} at 10 days to 90 000 at two years, whereas glial packing density increases from 30 000 cells mm^{-3} to 85 000 over the same period. The weight and volume of neurons also increase during the growth spurt and for some time thereafter, before levelling off. The pyramidal cells of cortical layer 5 have a mean volume of 460 μm^3 at birth, rising rapidly for 1–2 months and then slowly to 2505 μm^3 in the adult rat.

3.2   Neurogenesis

Development of the CNS is characterized by the migration of neurons from sites of origin in germinal centres in the wall of the early neural tube to their final positions. Initially, the wall of the neural tube is divisible into four zones: ventricular, subventricular, intermediate and marginal, with the cortical plate interspersed between them (Fig. 3–3).

Of these zones, the ventricular is the first to form alongside the lumen of the neural tube (or cerebral ventricle, as this part of it later becomes). On the outer aspect of the ventricular zone appears the marginal zone, with few cells and a continuous arrival and despatch of cell processes. The intermediate zone

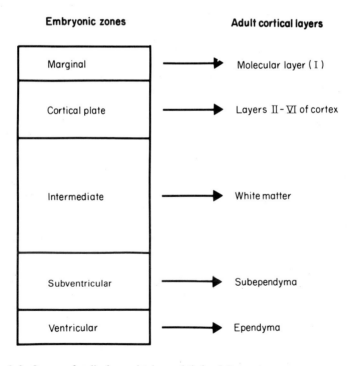

Fig. 3–3   Layers of wall of neural tube, and their adult counterparts.

becomes established between the ventricular and marginal zones, due to the arrival of postmitotic young neurons which send axons out into the marginal zone. Following this, further cells leave the ventricular zone and form a subventricular zone between the existing ventricular and intermediate zones. Further development involves elaboration of these existing zones, plus the cortical plate.

These zones are specific developmental structures because, with subsequent development, they either disappear or change out of all recognition (Fig. 3–3). The marginal zone eventually becomes the molecular layer of the cerebral cortex, with the cells of the cortical plate differentiating into the neurons of the remaining layers of the cortex. The intermediate zone becomes the white matter of the cortex, leaving the cells in the ventricular and subventricular zones to form the ependymal and subependymal cells, respectively.

The next step in understanding how the cerebral cortex develops is to consider the manner in which cells migrate within the cortex. In later gestation the major additions to the cortex are to its outer layers, necessitating a migration of cells through the cortical plate. The first formed cells reach the cortex rapidly, but the later cells with their longer migratory pathways take longer. Of the various ways in which cells may find their way to their final locations, the dominant idea is that of Rakic, namely, that the differentiating neurons are guided to the surface of the cortex by using radially-oriented glial fibres as guides. These *radial glia* have processes extending from ventricular to pial surfaces, one or two glial processes aiding the migration of several neurons.

The final position of the developing neurons is a matter for speculation. The most likely possibilities are that it is dictated by interaction of the migrating cell with processes of other cells, or that the information governing it is built into the postmitotic cell in the ventricular zone.

3.3   Development of neuronal processes

In 1910 Harrison observed that, as the growing *axon* increases in length, it produces numerous branches. Furthermore, the tips of both the initial outgrowth and the branches consist of an enlargement from which amoeboid terminal filaments are repeatedly emitted and retracted. This enlargement is the growth cone, first described by Ramon y Cajal in the 1890s.

The *growth cone* has a typical appearance, no matter what species is examined (Fig. 3–4). It is irregularly shaped and frequently gives rise to filopodia, which are mobile extensions up to 20 μm in length. Each growth cone has 1–30 filopodia associated with it; the filopodia are in constant motion, extending and retracting at a rate of 6–10 μm per minute. The leading edge of the growth cone functions as a locomotory organelle, and is also the site of elongation of the growth cone with newly-formed membrane deposited in this region.

The axonal growth cone displays a characteristic set of organelles, including agranular endoplasmic reticulum, vacuoles, large (growth cone) vesicles, microfilaments, possibly a few microtubules, and a dense network of neurofilaments

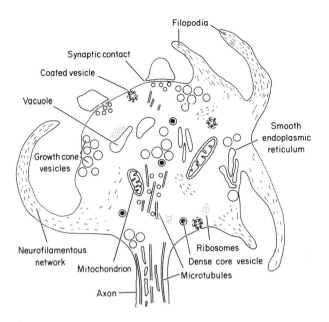

Fig. 3-4 Diagram of a growth cone to show its cytoplasmic organelles.

(Fig. 3-4). Mitochondria, dense-core vesicles and lysosomes also occur. The neurofilamentous network fills the periphery of the growth cone and penetrates the filopodia; it is attached to the inner surface of the surrounding membrane of the growth cone. Actin appears to be the principal constituent of the network, and may provide the structural and chemical basis needed for growth cone motility. The large vesicles and agranular endoplasmic reticulum are probably implicated in the provision of additional membrane for the growing tip.

Dendrites also have growth cones, and while these have much in common with the axonal variety, they can be distinguished by their population of large dense-core vesicles and ribosomes. They have a postsynaptic position, and new synapses are frequently made upon their filopodia.

Axonal growth cones persist until the appearance of the postsynaptic component of synapses, when they become altered by the loss of filopodia and the appearance of synaptic vesicles clustered in the vicinity of the postsynaptic density (§ 3.4).

The manner in which dendrites assume their final orientation differs in different parts of the dendritic tree. For instance, pyramidal cells of the cerebral cortex acquire their apical dendrites prior to the basal variety. Apical dendrites are initially random, and assume a radial orientation only with the migration of other neurons to more superficial positions. In the rat these events have been largely completed by birth. Twelve days later the dendritic tree is still poorly developed with a paucity of branching. This is rectified over the following two weeks by the peripheral extension and profuse branching of the dendrites. The result is that, by 30 days postnatal, the dendritic tree approaches its adult dimensions.

The final form of the dendritic tree is the result of a number of factors: extent of branching, length of the segments and their angles at the nodes. The last two factors may be under genetic influence, although the maturation of the tree as a whole is closely associated with the establishment of synaptic connections.

3.4   Synaptogenesis

Synapses result from a series of developmental events whereby growing axons make connections with processes of other neurons. Once viable connections are established, the growing axons with their growth cones develop into presynaptic terminals and the contacted regions of the other neurons become recognizable as postsynaptic sites. Debate about these events revolves round the mechanisms responsible for the direction of growth of the growth cone filopodia, and the nature of the initial contact.

Growing axons appear to move in characteristic directions without undue wandering or branching. Environmental factors play a role in this process, which does not however, restrict the axons to rigid pre-ordained routes. What is

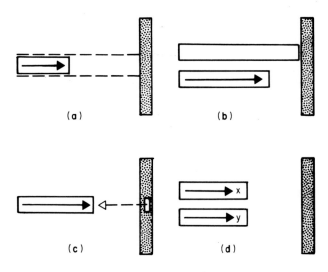

Fig. 3–5   Diagrams illustrating possible mechanisms of axonal growth. The horizontal blocks on the left represent growing axons, and the vertical blocks on the right postsynaptic sites. (**a**) Mechanical guidance; (**b**) contact guidance; (**c**) chemotaxis; (**d**) chemospecificity.

fascinating is that different axons exposed to the same environmental conditions respond differently by making different connections.

Various mechanisms for axonal growth and orientation have been postulated (Fig. 3–5). *Mechanical guidance* maintains that pre-established structural pathways (Fig. 3–5a, broken lines) link growing axons with their sites of termination, thereby restricting them to specific paths. An allied possibility is that once axons from a few cells have reached their terminations, later axons may reach the same region by *contact guidance* – using the original fibres as guides (Fig. 3–5b, upper axon). Alternatively, a chemical form of guidance may occur. *Chemotaxis* refers to the movement of cells along a chemical concentration gradient; the chemical diffuses from a source (Fig. 3–5c, in direction of arrow) and the responding cells detect local changes in concentration of the substance and alter their direction accordingly. *Chemospecificity* differs from chemotaxis, in that the chemical identification tag is thought to reside in the growing axon or neuron. Neurons would be distinguished by specific chemicals (Fig. 3–5d, X and Y), each with a preference for particular pathways.

Each of these mechanisms has its attractions and disadvantages. None of them can explain axonal orientation in its entirety, although each may

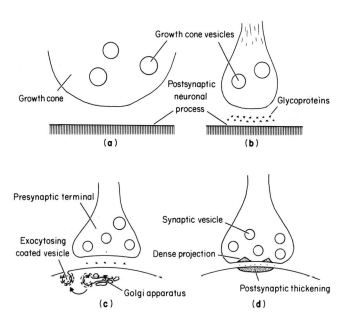

Fig. 3–6 Steps in the formation of synaptic contact. (a) Early (possibly transient) contact between leading edge of growth cone and postsynaptic neuronal process; (b) interneuronal recognition; (c) early development of postsynaptic thickening; (d) well-established synapse.

contribute to some aspect of it. It is also possible that the respective contributions of each of these individual mechanisms varies between synapses.

Before stable contacts between growing axons and postsynaptic neuronal processes are made, thousands of potential contact sites will have been bypassed. Mechanisms are required to recognize and bypass 'incorrect' contact points, and also to transform temporary 'correct' synapses into permanent ones. In some situations, transient synapses undoubtedly occur, although it is not clear how widespread this phenomenon is.

Initial contacts between growing axons and postsynaptic neuronal processes involve the outer coat material of the adjacent membranes. Interneuronal recognition is based on chemospecific glycoproteins. Once this has been accomplished, the specific thickenings characteristic of synaptic junctions begin to appear. It is far from clear what contributes to the formation of these specialized membrane thickenings, although coated vesicles have been put forward as candidates. The suggestion, as shown in Fig. 3–6, is that they bud off Golgi cisternae and contribute membrane to the neuronal surface in the vicinity of the contact zone. This could be accomplished if they were exocytosed in the vicinity of the developing synapse.

The next step in understanding how synapses are put together is to consider

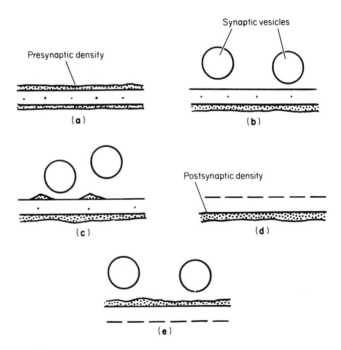

Fig. 3-7 Five alternative schemes by which synaptic junctions may develop.

the respective sequence of appearance of the pre- and postsynaptic membranes and the differential roles of the membrane thickenings and synaptic vesicles in the elaboration of the presynaptic contact area.

Figure 3–7 traces major ideas in this debate. In (a), both pre- and postsynaptic densities are present early in development, appearing as continuous plaques before the first synaptic vesicles appear. Later in development the plaques undergo gradual differentiation and focalization to produce the typical paramembranous densities of the adult synaptic junction (§ 4.2). An alternative is (b) with synaptic vesicles preceding presynaptic membrane thickenings. Another alternative is (c), in which increases in vesicle numbers and maturation of the paramembranous densities are more or less simultaneous events.

These possibilities assume that the pre- and postsynaptic membranes appear concurrently. This may not occur, as shown in (d), where the postsynaptic density appears as a well-established entity before the presynaptic region with its dense projections. The converse arrangement (e), whereby the presynaptic membrane appears prior to the postsynaptic is far less frequently encountered.

These diverse developmental patterns reflect the range of ways by which pre- and postsynaptic junctional elements establish their adult organization. It is not known whether a particular pattern characterizes a particular synaptic population, or whether similar synapses are put together in different ways under differing environmental pressures.

Once synapses have been established they increase dramatically in number during the growth spurt (§ 3.1). In rat cerebral cortex the most rapid increase in synaptic numbers occurs predominantly in the first two postnatal weeks. The precise period of rapid increase varies between different layers of the cerebral cortex. There may also be more than one period of rapid increase over the developmental period.

4 Synapses

4.1 Synaptic organization

Interesting as the synaptic *boutons* are, they failed to provide detailed understanding of the nature of the synaptic contacts between adjacent neurons. This had to await the advent of ultrastructural studies in the mid-1950s. Initial investigations, in the hands of people such as Eduardo De Robertis, Sanford Palay and George Palade, confirmed that the synaptic boutons are the enlarged axonal terminals while an extracellular cleft was clearly seen between the respective neurons. It soon became clear that the synaptic complex consists of three components: presynaptic terminal, cleft and postsynaptic process, the latter corresponding to the readily-seen dendritic spines (Fig. 1–4 and 4–1). Of perhaps greater interest were the 40 nm vesicular profiles (synaptic vesicles) within the presynaptic terminal, the size of the cleft (20 nm across) and the

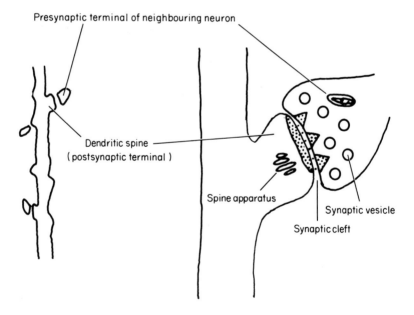

Fig. 4–1 Diagram to illustrate the transition from the light microscopic (left) to the electron microscopic (right) levels of synaptic analysis. The dendritic spine corresponds to the enlarged spines shown in the inset in Fig. 1–4.

overall polarization of the synapse due to the thickened membrane in the postsynaptic process (Figs 4–1 and 5–7). These observations solved two problems. The presence of an extracellular cleft showed in irrefutable terms what had been postulated for many years – that there is no cytoplasmic continuity between the neurons implicated in a synapse (§ 2.1). The sizes of the vesicles and cleft confirmed previous biophysical findings of Bernard Katz and co-workers that, at chemical synapses, the transmitter is carried by synaptic vesicles and liberated at the presynaptic membrane. More specifically, the synaptic vesicles are of the size and occupy the position expected of the quantal units of transmitter. This led to the vesicle hypothesis, according to which synaptic vesicles and quanta of chemical transmitter are equivalent; from this it follows that quantal release is equivalent to the release of the contents of one vesicle into the synaptic cleft. The validity of this hypothesis is discussed in Chapter 6.

4.2   Central synapses

4.2.1   Synaptic types

In the early 1960s two structurally different types of cortical synapses were described. The initial contribution to this endeavour was made by George Gray with his categorization of cortical synapses into types 1 and 2. This distinction was enunciated using osmium tetroxide (OsO_4)-fixed and phosphotungstic acid (PTA)-stained brain material. Type 1 synapses have prominent presynaptic dense projections, well-defined granular cleft material and an extensive post-synaptic thickening (Fig. 4–2a). By contrast, each of these features is less pronounced in type 2 synapses. In particular, the area of contact between the pre- and postsynaptic membrane thickenings in type 2 synapses is markedly less than in type 1 (Fig. 4–2a). Type 1 synapses frequently have an axodendritic location and type 2 an axosomatic one. Axodendritic synapses are usually formed between the terminal enlargements of axons and dendritic spines (Fig. 4–1); axosomatic synapses occur between axons and cell bodies.

This distinction between synaptic types has subsequently been extensively used in the literature and has, by now, become an integral part of synaptic terminology. In spite of this, it needs to be remembered that the fixation and staining schedule on which it is based, is no longer employed. The respective axodendritic and axosomatic locations of the two synaptic types is a generalization, which holds best in cerebral and cerebellar cortices. It is also a simplification, as there are far more synaptic types in existence than just axodendritic and axosomatic varieties. These include: dendrodendritic, axoaxonal and serial synapses (for presynaptic inhibition), even these being capable of further subdivision in different neuronal sites.

With the recognition of an ever-enlarging variety of morphological types has gone an awareness that an increasing number of chemical substances may serve as transmitter substances. Among these are acetylcholine, noradrenaline,

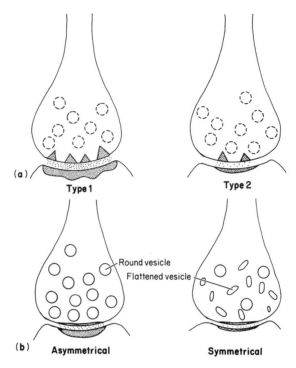

Fig. 4–2 Comparison of (**a**) types 1 and 2 synapses and (**b**) asymmetrical and symmetrical synapses. Note the presence of round vesicles in the asymmetrical synapse and flattened vesicles in the symmetrical one.

5-hydroxytryptamine, histamine, dopamine, γ-aminobutyric acid, glutamine, glycine, taurine and substance P. The relationship between a particular morphologically-identified synaptic type and a particular neurotransmitter is far from clear, and any one type may be associated with more than one transmitter.

Some progress has been made in this direction by correlating vesicle types with junction characteristics. It was noted by Koji Uchizono that, in aldehyde-fixed cerebellar cortex, synaptic vesicles in excitatory synapses are round, while those in inhibitory synapses are flattened. This observation holds for many other CNS situations as well and, while the rationale behind the flattening phenomenon has been ardently if inconclusively debated, the distinction has proved a helpful one. Alongside this observation, can be placed a complementary one, namely, that the Gray type 1 synapses are excitatory and Gray type 2 inhibitory. When it is realized that in routine aldehyde-OsO_4-fixed tissue Gray type 1 synapses are asymmetrical and Gray type 2 synapses symmetrical, we arrive at the equations: Gray type 1 = asymmetrical junction = round vesicles; and Gray type 2 = symmetrical junction = flattened vesicles (Fig. 4–2b).

These are generalizations, which do not hold in all neuronal circuits. Nevertheless, in many circumstances they are helpful ones and constitute an important, if preliminary, attempt at bridging the gap between morphological and functional realms. Unfortunately, the explanatory power of this model is decreasing as an increasing diversity of synaptic types – utilizing a wide range of excitatory and inhibitory transmitters – is found. The only definite relationship is that a preponderance of dense-core vesicles utilize noradrenaline as transmitter.

In the above discussion the terms asymmetrical and symmetrical refer to the appearance of synaptic membrane thickenings. In the asymmetrical variety the postsynaptic thickening is noticeably thicker than the corresponding presynaptic thickening; in the symmetrical variety the two are approximately equivalent (Figs 4–2b and 5–7). Excitatory synapses are those in which the passage of a nerve impulse lowers the membrane potential to form an excitatory postsynaptic potential. In inhibitory synapses a nerve impulse raises the membrane potential of the postsynaptic membrane. The result is an inhibitory postsynaptic potential. Excitation therefore, is the act of bringing a neuron to a state in which it is more likely to fire, whereas inhibition is the act of preventing a cell from firing.

4.2.2 Paramembranous densities

These are densities associated with the pre- and postsynaptic membranes. They are highlighted by the use of aldehyde-fixed, phosphotungstic acid-stained (E-PTA) material. The most prominent densities are the triangular-shaped dense projections in the presynaptic terminal and the postsynaptic thickening in the postsynaptic terminal (Figs 2–3 and 4–3). In transverse sections dense projections appear to be evenly distributed along the length of the presynaptic membrane (Fig. 4–3). Further light is cast on this arrangement when tangential sections, that is, sections at right-angles to transverse ones, are examined. Tangential sections through dense projections show that the projections have a triangular distribution (Fig. 4–3). Six spaces can be seen around each dense projection; these spaces probably correspond to the positions of synaptic vesicles, thereby ensuring that six vesicles can be accommodated around every one dense projection (Fig. 4–3).

The overall arrangement of the dense projections plus surrounding vesicular spaces is that of an orderly hexagonal grid, the *presynaptic vesicular grid* (Fig. 4–3). The focal points of this grid are provided by the dense projections, which are welded together by fine strands. The significance of this grid type of organization, first described by Gray and later elaborated by Konrad Akert, is that it allows one vesicle at a time to make contact with any one point on the presynaptic membrane. Since the synaptic vesicles, on reaching the presynaptic membrane, release their contents into the cleft, this form of grid organization introduces a means by which transmitter release can be controlled.

Important as the presynaptic vesicular grid is as a factor in transmitter release,

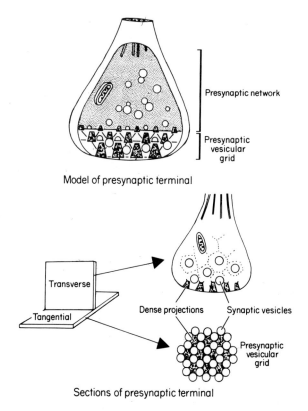

Fig. 4-3 The top diagram is a three-dimensional representation of a presynaptic terminal, highlighting the presynaptic vesicular grid, presynaptic network and synaptic vesicles. The lower diagrams depict transverse and tangential sections, the latter illustrating the presynaptic vesicular grid.

it is only present in the vicinity of the presynaptic membrane (Fig. 4–3). It extends for little more than 100 nm into the presynaptic terminal. Beyond this, such an orderly arrangement is not present; it is replaced by a more diffuse *presynaptic network* (Fig. 4–3). This is distributed throughout the terminal having connections with the dense projections and plasma membrane enveloping the terminal.

4.3 Neuromuscular junctions

One of the characteristic features of these junctions is the postsynaptic junctional folds (Fig. 4–4), with their regular spacing at 0.5–1.0 μm intervals. The presynaptic terminal is dominated by synaptic vesicles and, like the terminal

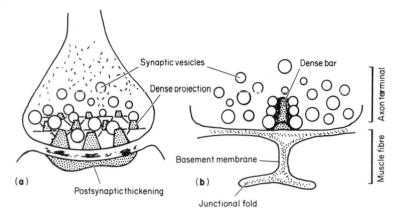

Fig. 4–4 Representations of (a) a central synapse, and (b) a neuromuscular junction, to show the dense projections and the dense bar, respectively, together with synaptic vesicles.

of central synapses, has presynaptic densities situated on the presynaptic membrane. Unlike the arrangement previously encountered, however, the densities occur as single dense bars facing the openings of the junctional folds. On either side of each bar is a row of synaptic vesicles (contrast a and b in Fig. 4–4).

Freeze fracture studies (§ 5.3) of the active zone of the presynaptic terminal and membrane have confirmed that the presynaptic densities are parallel bands running perpendicular to the long axis of the elongated nerve terminal. They probably represent specializations of the presynaptic membrane, enabling the vesicles to be brought into contact with the presynaptic membrane. Particles distributed regularly along the rims of the dense bars are thought to represent the attachment sites of synaptic vesicles to the presynaptic membrane. Because of the different arrangement of the presynaptic densities and synaptic vesicles in neuromuscular junctions and central synapses (Fig. 4–4) the packing of vesicle release sites differs in the two situations; they are four to eight times less densely-packed in neuromuscular synapses.

The typical presynaptic vesicular grid of central synapses is not present at neuromuscular junctions. The dense bars found in the latter are more akin to the bar type of synapses described in insect and some other invertebrate synapses. This type of synaptic arrangement leads to the interaction of a single active zone with two postsynaptic elements, unlike the one-to-one arrangement characteristic of central synapses (Fig. 4–4).

4.4 Electrical synapses

The organization of these synapses provides a low-resistance pathway between the neurons composing them. Electrotonic transmission occurs at these sites, which are characterized by minimal delay in synaptic transmission. This is a result of the absence of chemical mediation, and hence the lack of vesicle involvement in neurotransmission. Electrical synapses are not polarized, so that transmission can occur in two directions. These synapses are gap junctions, consisting of closely opposed pre- and postsynaptic membranes. The interval between them is about 2 nm, and in transverse section consists of a seven-layered arrangement: four dense lines alternating with three lighter ones. Two of the dense lines belong to each of the synaptic membranes. The 2 nm gap is extracellularly located, as it can be penetrated by tracer substances such as lanthanum salts. Electrical synapses are symmetrical and do not possess pre- and postsynaptic membrane thickenings.

Obliquely-sectioned electrical synapses have cross striations, while sections in the plane of the junctions reveal an array of closely-packed, hexagonal subunits. These can be delineated by lanthanum, suggesting they occupy the interneuronal gap. Freeze-fracture studies support this interpretation, with their demonstration of hexagonally-arranged membrane particles. Small channels, 2.5 nm in diameter, appear to cross from one neuron to the other within electrical synapses.

Electrical synapses are common in invertebrates and lower vertebrates, and occur infrequently in the mammalian nervous system including one of the trigeminal (fifth cranial nerve) nuclei and at the bipolar-ganglion cell junction of the retina.

5 Presynaptic Terminal

The presynaptic terminal refers to the enlarged termination of the axon (Figs 4–1 and 5–7), and corresponds to the *boutons terminaux* of light microscopy (§ 2.1). At the ultrastructural level it includes a specialized presynaptic membrane alongside the cleft, associated dense projections and a presynaptic vesicular grid (Fig. 4–4). Within the terminal cytoplasm are synaptic and coated vesicles, mitochondria, cisterns, vacuoles, a microfilamentous presynaptic network and possibly microtubules. Under appropriate circumstances vesicle attachment sites may also be present at the presynaptic membrane (Fig. 5–1).

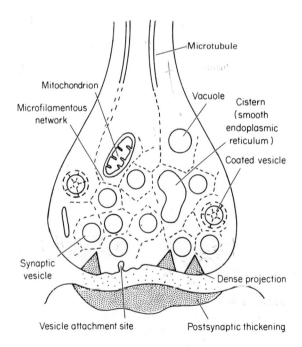

Fig. 5–1 The presynaptic terminal of a central synapse, depicting its major components. These components are highlighted by different fixation and staining techniques, and are shown together to give an impression of the terminal as an integrated unit.

5.1   Microfilamentous network

Proteins with actomyosin-like, actin-like and myosin-like properties are present in brain tissue. As these are the contractile proteins of muscle, it follows that contractile filaments are present within nervous tissue. These proteins are widely distributed throughout the brain and occur in most parts of neurons. Evidence favouring their location in presynaptic terminals comes from the finding of actomyosin in synaptosomes (terminals that have been separated from the axon proper by homogenization and centrifugation procedures). High actin levels have also been reported in cultures of sympathetic ganglia, and in developing and adult chick brain.

When synaptosomes are subfractionated, the synaptic vesicles released are primarily associated with a myosin-like protein and the membrane fractions with an actin-like protein. Using these data it has been speculated that the actin of the presynaptic terminal membrane reacts with the myosin of synaptic vesicles to draw the latter towards the presynaptic membrane. At the membrane, the actin and myosin may be implicated in opening the synaptic vesicles and presynaptic membrane (in response to the influx of calcium) and releasing transmitter into the cleft.

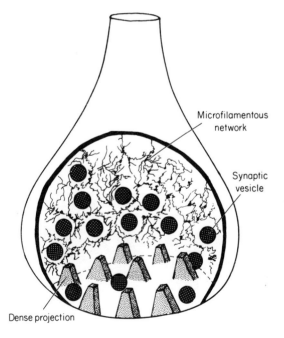

Microfilamentous
network

Synaptic
vesicle

Dense projection

Fig. 5–2   Diagrammatic representation of the distribution of the HMM-stained microfilamentous network throughout the presynaptic terminal.

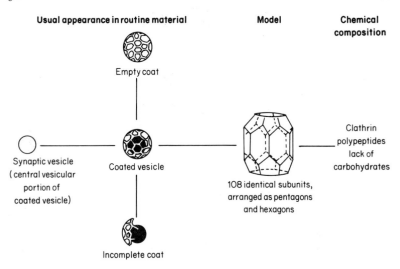

Fig. 5–3 Summary of the structure and chemical composition of coated vesicles.

Using the technique of heavy meromyosin (HMM) labelling, actin-like filaments can be visualized in presynaptic terminals. They form a dense network surrounding mitochondria and synaptic vesicles, and are possibly anchored at various points to the inner surface of the terminal membrane and dense projections (Fig. 5–2). This actin microfilamentous network closely resembles the presynaptic network (§ 4.2), suggesting that the network is widely distributed throughout presynaptic terminals.

Actin is associated with microfilaments. These are about 6 nm in diameter; they have a subunit molecular weight of 46 000 and consititute 10–15% of the total protein in nervous tissue (compared with 25% in striated muscle). Other filaments found in nervous tissues are brain intermediate filaments (neuro-filaments), with a diameter of approximately 10 nm and a molecular weight of 51 000.

5.2   Coated vesicles

These consist of a central vesicle (an ordinary synaptic vesicle) enclosed within a coat (or basket) having a dense spiny arrangement (Fig. 5–3). Each coat is composed of regular pentagons and hexagons with sides of equal length. Using a fractionation scheme to obtain a relatively pure sample of coated vesicles, the proteins of the coat can be elucidated. One protein species, *clathrin*, has a molecular weight of 180 000 and is located on the vesicle surface. It accounts for 40–70% of the total vesicle protein, the remainder being made up of proteins with molecular weights of 125 000 and 55 000.

Coated vesicles occur widely in biological material and are involved in the uptake and transport of proteins and enzymes. They probably also play a role in the infolding of cell membranes, a role scrutinized by neurobiologists in an attempt to understand the significance of coated vesicles for synaptic function.

According to the vesicle hypothesis (Chapter 6) synaptic vesicles loaded with neurotransmitter arrive at the presynaptic membrane and release transmitter into the cleft. Following irreversible exocytosis, they become incorporated into the presynaptic membrane (Fig. 5–4). The vesicle membrane passes 'through' the plasma membrane of the presynaptic terminal, reaching a site away from the cleft region, where it is returned to the interior of the terminal by endocytosis. This recapturing process is brought about by coating of the invaginated membrane. The coated invagination then breaks off to become a typical coated vesicle which, in turn, gradually sheds its coat to form a synaptic vesicle or merges with other coated vesicles to give rise to a vacuole or cistern (Fig. 5–4). Synaptic vesicles subsequently bud-off the cisterns.

Coated vesicles may also help reduce the calcium level in the terminal following neurotransmitter release. This possibility is based on their ability to

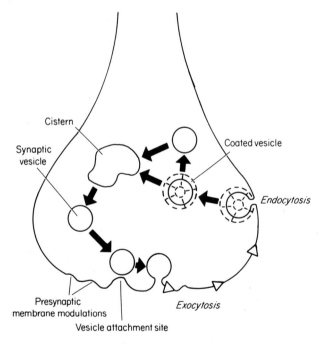

Fig. 5–4 Illustration of the presumed way in which membrane is recycled through the presynaptic terminal. The black arrows show the direction in which membrane travels, assuming that exocytosis and endocytosis occur at the locations shown. The open arrowheads depict the movement of vesicle membrane within the terminal membrane following exocytosis and as a prelude to endocytosis.

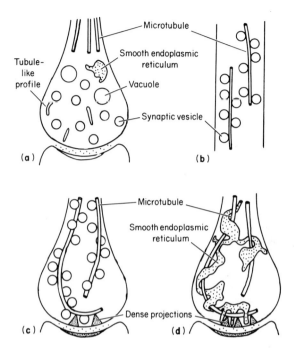

Fig. 5-5   Models of the presynaptic terminal.

sequester calcium ions, and on the fact that neurotransmitter release is triggered by calcium influx. Such a role would prevent uncontrolled exocytosis. Calcium uptake by coated vesicles may also be necessary for the fusion of coated vesicle membranes with that of other organelle membranes.

5.3   Microtubular system

Microtubules are conventionally depicted terminating at the junction of the axon proper and its presynaptic enlargement (Fig. 5–5a). Along the axon there is a close interrelationship between synaptic vesicles and microtubules with, in some instances, five vesicles occurring in a rosette arrangement around single microtubules. There may also be structural links between the vesicles and microtubules (Fig. 5–5b). Besides microtubules, there is a range of tubular-type inclusion such as vacuoles, cisternae, tubule-like profiles, and microtubule-smooth endoplasmic reticulum complexes.

Microtubules are characterized by the presence of tubulin which has a molecular weight of 110 000. It consists of two subunits, α and β-tubulin, with 53 000 and 55 000 molecular weights respectively. Approximately 10–20% of the total protein of developing brain is in the form of soluble tubulin.

Microtubules are responsible for the rapid transport of many intracellular particles, and in neurons take part in the axoplasmic transport of vesicles, mitochondria and protein along the axon from the cell body of the nerve terminal. Microtubules are also involved in excitation-secretion coupling mechanisms, for instance, the release of insulin and transmitter substances. Tubulin may account for as much as 25% of the soluble protein of synaptosomes, and is a major component of the postsynaptic thickening. Synaptosomal tubulin appears to have an unusual subunit arrangement. It has been suggested these results could be due to contamination of the synaptosomal fractions by a tubulin-like polypeptide from the postsynaptic thickening.

Typically, microtubules are not seen in the presynaptic terminal of central synapses. They have been identified in synaptosomes incubated at room temperature, and in presynaptic terminals when previously-damaged material is treated with albumin or distilled water prior to fixation. Microtubules traverse the terminal and end at dense projections (Fig. 5–5c). These presynaptic microtubules have vesicles distributed along their length, like microtubule-vesicle associations in axons (cf. Fig. 5–5 b and c). It has also been claimed that cisternae of the smooth endoplasmic reticulum may be similarly wound around these microtubules (Fig. 5–5d).

It is feasible that these terminal microtubules are axonal microtubules that have been pulled down from the axon during preparation of the material. If, however, they are *in situ* microtubules, they may be responsible for drawing vesicles to the region of the presynaptic membrane. Should this be so, the relationship between the microtubules and microfilamentous network requires clarification. Alternatively, the synaptic vesicles could represent broken down smooth endoplasmic reticulum. If this is the case, current ideas regarding synaptic organization, endocytosis-exocytosis of vesicle membrane and membrane recycling at the presynaptic terminal will have to be re-assessed (Chapter 6).

5.4   Vesicle-membrane relationships

A missing element from this account of synaptic organization is the relationship between synaptic vesicles and the presynaptic membrane. Figure 5–4 illustrates the conventional picture of the vesicle fusing with the presynaptic membrane, although doubt remains about the fate of the vesicle itself. Thin-sectioned material is limited in the information it is capable of providing on the intimate association between vesicles and the presynaptic membrane, and for help in this direction recourse to freeze-fracture studies is essential.

Freeze-fracture of biological material causes unit membranes to split so that the internal surfaces of both leaflets are exposed. The presynaptic membrane is viewed either as the outer face of its inner leaflet (PF, P face) or as the inner face of its outer leaflet (EF, E face).

The presynaptic area in freeze-fracture material is characterized by an accumulation of intramembranous particles and the aggregation of 20 nm profiles which appear as protuberances or pits depending on the membrane face examined (Fig. 5–6). Protuberances are seen on inspection of the inner face of

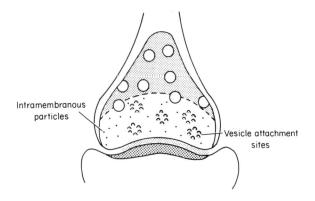

Intramembranous
particles

Vesicle attachment
sites

Fig. 5–6 Diagrammatic representation of the major features characterizing the presynaptic area in freeze-fractured central synapses.

the outer leaflet (EF), and pits on the corresponding outer face of the inner leaflet (PF). In other words, protuberances are seen when a junction is viewed from the presynaptic cytoplasmic side, and pits when examined from the extracellular space of the cleft. When these protuberances/pits are clearly seen, they appear in groups and on some occasions have a hexagonal arrangement (Fig. 5–6). Of particular interest is their spacing from one another: 40–50 nm. This corresponds to the spacing of synaptic vesicles around dense projections in the presynaptic vesicular grid (Fig. 4–3). Accordingly, it has been postulated that they serve as sites for the attachment of vesicles to the presynaptic membrane, hence their name, vesicle attachment sites (VAS).

Once a vesicle becomes attached to a VAS, the contiguous membranes fuse, thereby opening a channel for the passage of the transmitter substance from the vesicle and through the presynaptic membrane. The membranes then reseal, allowing the vesicle to move back into the terminal (reversible exocytosis) or the vesicle membrane becomes incorporated into the terminal membrane and the vesicle disappears (irreversible exocytosis).

Although VAS appear to be specific sites at which vesicles adhere to the presynaptic membrane, it is important to look for evidence other than the purely morphological. One useful avenue is to compare the appearance of anaesthetized with unanaesthetized terminals. Most experimental animals are first anaesthetized with sodium pentobarbitone (Nembutal) and it has recently become clear that this alters both the structure and the functioning of CNS synapses. In freeze-fracture and thin-sectioned material, VAS are far more frequent and clearly defined in unanaesthetized material than following the use of an anaesthetic. Besides this, in freeze-fracture material there are more VAS with crater-like appearances at their apices (open-type VAS). It has been suggested that these VAS represent vesicles that have fused with the presynaptic membrane, so that fluctuations in their numbers probably correspond to the quantal release of synaptic transmitter substances.

Another approach to the significance of VAS is provided by their response to incubation in high-potassium media and to electrical stimulation. Incubation of the sea lamprey's spinal cord in a high-potassium plus calcium medium results in a marked increase in the numbers of VAS per synaptic profile. By contrast, replacement of calcium by magnesium in the medium fails to replicate this increase in VAS numbers, pointing to the intimate association between functioning synapses, which require the presence of calcium, and VAS sites. This association is further underlined by an increase in a high-postassium plus calcium medium. When nervous tissue is electrically stimulated, a similar increase in the overall number of VAS, as well as in the percentage of the open-type variety, occurs in some situations.

There are strong grounds for believing, therefore, that a correlation exists between synaptic functioning and the presence of VAS. Similar results have been forthcoming from experiments on frog neuromuscular junctions, although most studies suffer from a reliance on fairly slow fixation procedures. As these procedures are much slower than the processes involved in neurotransmission, precise details of the membrane cycling sequence of events are obscured. To overcome this obstacle, John Heuser and Thomas Reese in the latter part of the 1970s employed a very rapid method of freezing tissue. They dispensed with ordinary fixation procedures and were able to detect structural changes occurring within a small fraction of a millisecond.

Using a combination of chemical and quick-freezing techniques, it appears that the exocytotic-endocytotic cycling mechanism is an integral part of neurotransmitter release. It is also possible to distinguish between exocytotic and endocytotic sites in freeze-fracture material. This suggests that during endocytosis specific components of the synaptic vesicle membranes are preserved and can, presumably, be re-utilized in new synaptic vesicles (Fig. 5–4).

5.5   Models of the presynaptic terminal

Some of the wide range of organelles and profiles encountered in the presynaptic terminal of central synapses are shown in Figs 5–1 and 5–7. At present it is difficult to formulate any one satisfactory model of the presynaptic terminal, because of the multiplicity of techniques used to demonstrate the many terminal profiles. Two principles require consideration: no constituent of the terminal can be considered in isolation from other constituents; the constituents of the terminal are highly labile.

Figure 5–5 presents a composite model of the terminal, with four possible models representing different aspects of the terminal's organization. A microfilamentous network is probably implicated in drawing vesicles into the vesicular grid, the arrangement of which imposes limitations on where the vesicles make contact with the presynaptic membrane. This constitutes a morphological counterpart to quantal neurotransmission. Membrane turnover is accomplished via exocytotic and endocytotic sites as membrane moves between various terminal compartments. It may be that a microtubule system provides a long-term mechanism for producing vesicles, with a microfilamentous system providing the structural framework for a short-term membrane retrieval mechanism.

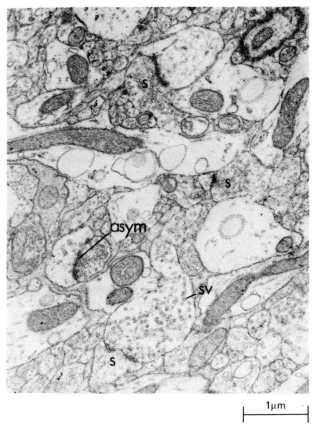

1μm

Fig. 5-7 Electron micrograph of synapses in rat cerebral cortex. Synapses (s) are seen with synaptic vesicles (sv) in their presynaptic terminals. Most synapses have asymmetrical (asym) thickenings.

6 Vesicle Hypothesis

This hypothesis has provided the framework for most contemporary thinking about synaptic organization, as a result of which its influence on synaptic concepts has been immense. In previous chapters it has been necessary to refer repeatedly to the hypothesis, on acount of its wide-ranging explanatory properties. Nevertheless, its validity has been questioned by various workers, and because of its significance for synaptic thinking, the contending arguments require close attention.

6.1 Nature of the vesicle hypothesis

The demonstration that transmitter substances are released in discrete quantal packages, coupled with ultrastructural observations of presynaptically located synaptic vesicles, set the scene for the vesicle hypothesis (§ 4.1). According to this, transmitter substances are stored within synaptic vesicles and conveyed by them to the presynaptic membrane. In its simplest form, this hypothesis states that the synaptic vesicle and quantum of chemical transmitter are equivalent (Fig. 6–1), from which it follows that quantal release is equivalent to the release of the contents of one vesicle into the synaptic cleft.

The close correspondence between the ultrastructural characteristics of the subcellular particles as predicted by the quantal theory and the actual vesicles observed by electron microscopy was sufficient to ensure rapid adoption of the

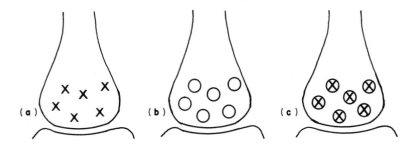

Fig. 6–1 Diagrams to illustrate relationship between quantal theory of neurotransmission and vesicle hypothesis. In (a) X represents quantal packets of transmitter; (b) depicts the synaptic vesicles, as seen in electron micrographs; (c) illustrates the vesicle hypothesis in its simple form, in which quanta and vesicles are equated.

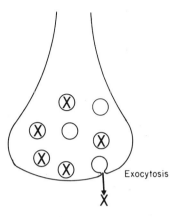

Fig. 6–2 In terms of the vesicle hypothesis, transmitter is released from the presynaptic terminal by exocytosis. The transmitter is represented by X.

idea by an overwhelming majority of synaptologists. It was postulated that when vesicles, with their content of transmitter, touch the presynaptic membrane at critical points, the transmitter is released by exocytosis (Fig. 6–2). Nerve stimulation would be expected to increase the probability of contact and thus of transmitter release. This was regarded as a satisfactory explanation of the occurrence of miniature end-plate potentials (mepp) and of the quantal character of the evoked end-plate potential (epp). It also explained how quanta are formed and stored in the presynaptic terminal for ready release.

This hypothesis received considerable support from early subcellular fractionation studies of cholinergic neurons, which demonstrated the preferential localization within synaptosomes derived from brain tissue of acetylcholine (ACh) and the enzymes of the ACh system, acetylcholinesterase and choline-acetyltransferase. Furthermore, synaptic vesicles isolated from synaptosomes have the highest specific concentration of ACh.

These results demonstrated that the relationship between synaptic vesicles and ACh is a close, and perhaps even a direct, one. Not surprisingly, the conclusion was reached that synaptic vesicles actually correspond to the quanta of transmitter, a necessary equation for the vesicle hypothesis (Fig. 6–1).

Although this represents a simple solution to the problem of neurotransmission, it leaves unanswered certain basic questions, the main one of which concerns the *mechanism* of transmitter release. The vesicle hypothesis is based on the assumption that transmitter is released from the presynaptic terminal by exocytosis (Fig. 6–2). Numerous difficulties have been encountered, however, in unequivocally demonstrating that this is the principal release mechanism, and these difficulties eventually led to a questioning of exocytosis as the release mechanism. This questioning has, in turn, led to a re-opening of the vesicle-quantum relationship issue.

An allied difficulty has been the cytoplasmic as well as vesicular location of ACh in the presynaptic terminal. Subcellular fractionation studies point to the existence of cytoplasmic ('free'; extravesicular) ACh (Fig. 6–3), of which no account is taken by the vesicle hypothesis. In response to this, two alternatives have been put forward: either cytoplasmic ACh is taken up by vesicles prior to its release by exocytosis, or it is released directly from the cytoplasm without vesicular intervention. The latter could be accomplished by the opening of a channel in the presynaptic membrane; such a 'membrane-gate' mechanism has been viewed as an alternative to the vesicle hypothesis (Fig. 6–3).

Whatever the validity of the vesicle hypothesis, the existence of synaptic vesicles and quanta is not seriously in dispute. The point of contention is the nature of the relationship (if any) between them.

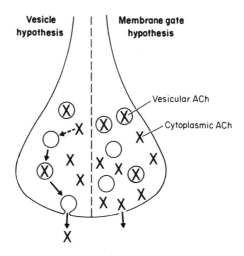

Fig. 6–3 Comparison of the demands of the vesicle hypothesis and a membrane-gate hypothesis.

6.2   Status of the vesicle hypothesis

6.2.1   Morphological evidence

A relationship between synaptic vesicle numbers and neurotransmitter levels is suggested by stimulation experiments in which severe fatigue of transmitter release is associated with reduction in vesicle numbers. Recovery from fatigue is accompanied by a reappearance of vesicles and the attainment of normal vesicle numbers. When this experimental system is coupled, in the neuromuscular junction, with the use of horseradish peroxidase (HRP) as a cytochemical tracer, it is possible to follow the passage of vesicle membrane through the presynaptic terminal (Fig. 5–5). The extracellular HRP is taken into the terminal by endocytosis following stimulation; it then passes through the various membrane compartments of the terminal and is released into the cleft by exocytosis. This is demonstrated by the appearance of large numbers of vesicle attachment sites (VAS) at the presynaptic membrane when preparations are stimulated at the moment of aldehyde fixation (§ 5.3).

A limitation of this model is the slow speed with which aldehyde fixation arrests synaptic function. As a result it is not possible to be sure that vesicle exocytosis is occurring at the exact moment of transmitter release, thereby precluding any correlation of the number of discharged vesicles with the number of quanta released.

To overcome these problems Heuser developed a quick-freezing technique which, at the neuromuscular junction, enables a single shock to be delivered to the nerve, which is frozen at the peak of the postsynaptic end-plate potential produced. When examined in the electron microscope, the number of vesicles caught in the act of discharge and the number of quanta that would have produced an end-plate potential of that amplitude can be compared. From this, Heuser considers that synaptic vesicle exocytosis occurs at precisely the same moment as transmitter release, with one vesicle discharged for each quantum released – as predicted by the vesicle hypothesis.

In order to stimulate the transmitter release in this experiment, the drug 4-aminopyridine is employed. This produces an abnormally high discharge, and hence an unusually large number of exocytotic vesicles. This facilitates quantitative analysis of transmitter release because 4-aminopyridine blocks potassium channels, thereby allowing the entry of large amounts of calcium. The resulting end-plate response is increased 50–100 fold by the presence of 1 mM of the drug.

Apart from the non-physiological nature of this model, a major criticism is that the exocytotic phenomena may be connected with processes *following*, rather than accompanying, transmitter release. If so, they would not be *responsible for* transmitter release, which would have occurred prior to the appearance of the membrane modulations. This interpretation is based on a 3 msec delay in the appearance of presynaptic membrane modulations following stimulation. This is longer than the average synaptic delay (0.75 msec) at neuromuscular junctions, even allowing a further 1 msec for transmission down the nerve.

6.2.2   Biochemical evidence

The crux of objections to the vesicle hypothesis is the existence of cytoplasmic ACh. Approximately 50% of terminal ACh exists in synaptic vesicles at a concentration of 150 mM. The remaining 50% is cytoplasmically located, at a concentration of 20–30 mM. The question is whether stimulation of the nerve leads to the release of vesicular or cytoplasmic ACh.

The electric organ of *Torpedo* is a useful experimental model for transmitter investigations, as it contains very high levels of ACh and is morphologically analogous to the neuromuscular junction. When physiologically stimulated, some workers claim there is preferential release of cytoplasmic ACh (Fig. 6–3). The depletion and turn-over of cytoplasmic ACh is not accompanied by any detectable transfer to vesicular ACh, which remains unchanged by the stimulation. There is no radioactive exchange into the vesicles, as would be expected had they been refilled with ACh.

A further step in this argument is that the most recently synthesized ACh is located in the cytoplasm (Fig. 6–4). This, together with the cytoplasmic location of the enzyme for synthesizing ACh, choline acetyltransferase, has been taken to suggest that the ACh released on stimulation is of the recently synthesized variety and comes directly from the terminal cytoplasm.

This interpretation leaves little room for a vesicular role in transmitter release, although a frequently encountered suggestion is that they provide a reserve pool of ACh to replenish the cytoplasmic compartment when required (Fig. 6–4). It has also been proposed that vesicle exocytosis is a means of disposing of excess calcium from the presynaptic terminal, since about 30 times more calcium ions penetrate into the terminal than transmitter molecules leave it.

Such a major role for cytoplasmic ACh is by no means generally accepted by biochemists. In particular, Victor Whittaker, who has made a major contribution to an understanding of synaptic biochemistry through the development of subcellular fractionation techniques, contends that much of the cytoplasmic ACh is, in fact, vesicular in location.

In Whittaker's original subfractionation of synaptosomes he described one

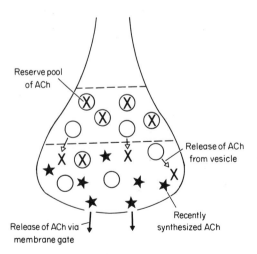

Fig. 6–4   Model of the presynaptic terminal, in which recently synthesized ACh is cytoplasmically located and synaptic vesicles represent a reserve pool of ACh.

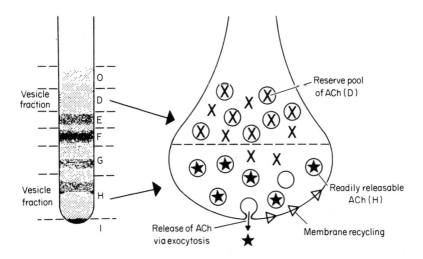

Fig. 6–5 Alternative model to that shown in Fig. 6–4. On the left, D and H represent vesicle fractions; these correspond respectively to the storage and readily releasable vesicles depicted in the presynaptic terminal on the right.

vesicle fraction (D), the remaining fractions consisting of membrane and synaptosomal fragments (Fig. 6–5). Whittaker and co-workers now describe an additional, denser vesicle fraction (H) which, according to them, displays the characteristics others ascribe to cytoplasmic ACh. From this it follows that newly synthesized ACh plus adenosine triphosphate (ATP), are preferentially located in the H vesicles. The ability of the H vesicles to take up newly synthesized transmitter is linked by these workers to the loss of pre-existing transmitter stocks. It is further argued that the H vesicles are close to the presynaptic membrane, are 25% smaller than the more proximally situated D vesicles, and hence are the vesicles being recycled (Fig. 6–5). Continued stimulation recruits more and more D vesicles into the H vesicular pool.

According to this scheme, the D vesicles serve as storage sites of transmitter, whereas the H vesicles represent the readily releasable transmitter (Fig. 6–5). This H subfraction of vesicles corresponds to the membrane channel of terminal models dependent on a non-vesicular release mechanism (§ 6.3).

6.3   Membrane-gate hypothesis

For those who dispense with the vesicle hypothesis an alternative means of liberating the transmitter from the presynaptic terminal must be found. Some form of membrane channel (gate) is the most highly favoured alternative (Fig. 6–3), although there is no specific evidence in its favour. Its plausibility in the presynaptic terminal stems from the existence in the postsynaptic process of a channel that allows sodium ions to move through membrane and bring about miniature end-plate potentials of constant amplitude.

In an attempt to delineate further a membrane-gating form of release mechanism, Maurice Israel applies the term, operator, to the functional unit responsible for ACh release. These operators, located at the presynaptic membrane, would be able to bind a given amount of cytoplasmic ACh in a saturable and reversible manner and subsequently, when triggered by calcium entry, deliver it into the synaptic cleft. Because of their close proximity to the presynaptic membrane, operators – it is hypothesized – would be preferentially fed by newly-synthesized ACh. The nature of these operators is speculative; they may be operative vesicles attached to the membrane, saturable gates or carrier proteins able to bind fixed amounts of ACh (Fig. 6–6).

These possibilities fit the expectations of a very dynamic release mechanism, although they have not as yet been subject to experimental testing. As they stand, they owe little to morphological concepts, and more work in this direction is required.

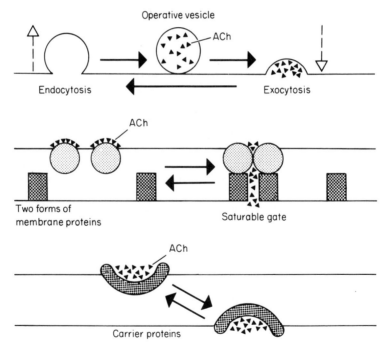

Fig. 6–6   Three possible forms of an ACh releasing operator mechanism. (a) Operative vesicle; (b) saturable gate; (c) carrier protein. (Based on ISRAEL *et al.*, 1979.)

6.4 Conclusions

Verification of the vesicle hypothesis requires that four conditions be met. These are: (*i*) ACh should be present in synaptic vesicles; (*ii*) nerve stimulation should preferentially release vesicular ACh prior to that of other terminal compartments; (*iii*) most of the releasable ACh should be in quanta; (*iv*) contact between vesicles and the presynaptic membrane should release vesicular ACh by exocytosis.

Of these conditions there is no doubt that (*i*) is met, and little doubt that (*iii*) and (*iv*) are. By far the most contentious is (*ii*).

Neurochemical evidence points definitively towards synaptic vesicles containing ACh. Unfortunately the CNS, in which measurements of the ACh content of vesicles are known, lacks a satisfactory estimate of the ACh content of quanta. Conversely neuromuscular junctions, which lend themselves to reliable estimates of the ACh content of quanta, are poor models for measurements of vesicle ACh content.

ACh is generally released in quantal form, although there are probably a few exceptions to this rule. Under some conditions non-quantal release may take place, but it is highly unlikely that fully-developed synaptic transmission occurs in the absence of synaptic vesicles. Morphological approaches, by themselves, cannot provide unequivocal evidence that synaptic vesicles fusing with the presynaptic membrane contain ACh; neither can they distinguish between those vesicles that do or do not contain transmitter.

It is unclear whether cytoplasmic ACh is a 'real' compartment or is partly derived from vesicular ACh. Unfortunately cytoplasmic ACh levels represent the difference between the total tissue content of ACh and the amount of ACh remaining after tissue homogenization. As a consequence, the experimental conditions employed and the purity of the fractions obtained are critical factors, since these affect the amount of ACh released from synaptic vesicles during preparative procedures.

Whittaker's concept of a H subfraction of vesicles is probably legitimate, although it is likely to contain some cytoplasm and hence some cytoplasmically-located ACh. It is also debatable whether the H subfraction is entirely vesicular in composition. This is a crucial issue to the vesicle hypothesis debate.

The vesicle hypothesis in its simple form (Fig. 6–1) appears untenable, as the vesicles of the presynaptic terminal are probably not the homogeneous entities once believed. The debate then becomes whether a modified version of this hypothesis or some form of membrane-gating alternative better fits the available data. Both alternatives are obliged to find an adequate explanation for the existence of synaptic vesicles. From a morphologist's standpoint a hypothesis incorporating proximal storage vesicles and distal vesicles actively involved in transmitter release and membrane recycling (Fig. 6–5) is the most acceptable current postulate.

Even a modified version of the vesicle hypothesis raises many intriguing questions. Among these are: the manner in which transmitter is transferred from the terminal cytoplasm to the vesicles; the means by which synaptic vesicles move within the terminal; the factors that determine the uniformity of vesicle size; the extent to which local membrane recycling occurs in the terminal; and the relationship between terminal and axonal processes.

7 Neural Plasticity

Functional regeneration within the mammalian CNS has been vigorously and inconclusively debated for many years. Despite over a century of intensive research, information essential to the understanding of the mechanisms underlying neural plasticity is incomplete. Certain earlier investigators were deceived by the degree of regeneration possible in the peripheral nervous system; their false reports of equally extensive CNS regeneration proved a fruitless experimental cul-de-sac. Cajal however, was not so easily misled and, in the late 1920s, concluded pessimistically: 'In adult centres the nerve paths are something fixed, ended, immutable. Everything may die, nothing may be regenerated'.

Possible factors responsible for such abortive CNS regeneration include absence of supportive elements and presence of either scar tissue or abnormal synapses. Efforts in the 1940s and 1950s to reduce scar tissue formation following spinal cord lesions were surprisingly successful, and prompted a reappraisal of the feasibility of axonal regeneration in adult CNS. Over the last two decades development of increasingly refined research tools has led to the view that the mammalian CNS is partially able to rebuild itself following lesions.

7.1 Plasticity concepts

Evidence suggests that many neurons in the CNS can re-organize their synaptic connections to form entirely new ones in response to lesions. This is the process of *reactive synaptogenesis*: a reaction to some stimulus, rather than part of the normal developmental process. Deafferentation (cutting incoming nerve fibres) elicits nearby undamaged fibres to grow and form new synaptic connections.

The most likely mechanism responsible for reactive synaptogenesis is *axonal sprouting*, which describes the sprouting of intact remaining neuronal afferent fibres into areas of partial neuronal deafferentation. These axonal sprouts may be produced in a variety of ways. In *collateral sprouting* axonal collaterals grow more extensively than normal and make contact with the denervated target cell either at a new postsynaptic site or at the original one (Fig. 7–1a). An alternative is *paraterminal sprouting*, the production of new terminals from existing axon terminals; these may subsequently form new synapses adjacent to degenerating ones (Fig. 7–1b).

Collateral sprouting is most effective when the lesion spares part of the innervation, leaving that spared part to compensate for the lost connections through expansion of its terminal field. The vacated synapses will be replaced by the remaining axons of the same pathway, having the same functional characteristics

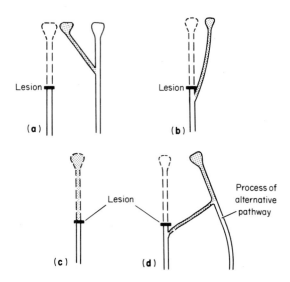

Fig. 7-1 Examples of (**a**) collateral sprouting, (**b**) paraterminal sprouting, (**c**) true regeneration, (**d**) use of previously unused pathway. The processes in broken lines are degenerating; the stippled processes are sprouting or regenerating.

as the lost ones (Fig. 7-1a). Collateral sprouting has been demonstrated in the hippocampus, spinal cord, visual cortex and sympathetic system. Lack of specificity in the sprouting process may sometimes produce anomalous connections resulting, for example, in spasticity after spinal cord lesions.

True regeneration of severed axons may occur in the CNS, resulting in regrowth of sprouting fibres back to their target sites (Fig. 7-1c). Evidence in favour of this phenomenon has been found in the hypothalamo-hypophyseal tract, olfactory bulb and spinal cord of adult rats. Partial regeneration can also be effective due to an increased functional efficiency of the few regenerated fibres.

Yet another possible sprouting mechanism involves the use of a *previously unused pathway*. This implies that an alternative intact pathway, which normally does not have the same function as the lesioned pathway, mediates that function through a re-adjustment of neural connections. A possible means of accomplishing this is shown in Fig. 7-1d, in which information is transferred from the lesioned system onto the intact one. At present there is little evidence for this mechanism.

7.2 Collateral sprouting

The most thorough investigations of this process have utilized the hippocampal dentate gyrus and septum.

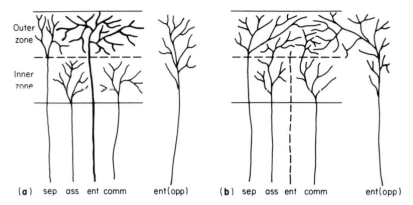

Fig. 7-2 In (a) the various inputs to the dentate gyrus are shown; association (ass.), commissural (comm.), entorhinal (ent.) of the same and opposite (opp.) sides, and septal (sep) fibres. In (b) the response shown is to degeneration of the entorhinal fibres of the same side.

7.2.1 Dentate gyrus

As shown in Fig. 7-2a, the molecular layer of the dentate gyrus is subdivided into inner and outer zones. The inner zone receives inputs from the pyramidal cells of the same (association fibres) and opposite (commissural fibres) sides, while the outer zone is innervated by the entorhinal cortex (entorhinal fibres) of the same side and by septal fibres. These four inputs are joined by a fifth (entorhinal of the opposite side) which terminates adjacent to the molecular layer.

Removal of the entorhinal cortex cuts off the entorhinal input of the same side, and is followed by sprouting of the remaining four afferents. These are depicted in Fig. 7-2b, showing that the association and commissural projections spread outwards, the septal fibres proliferate, and the entorhinal fibres of the opposite side make their way into the outer region of the molecular layer. Neurophysiological evidence for the establishment of synaptic contacts within certain of these rearranged systems has been obtained. The normal density of synapses in the molecular layer drops from 35 to 5 per 100 μm^2 within two days of a lesion, to return to normal by 240 days postlesion. Approximately 80% of the original synapses are reformed through reinnervation from the opposite side. The majority of new synapses are probably formed *de novo*; if this is so, the adult CNS has the capacity to carry out all necessary steps involved in synaptogenesis.

7.2.2 Septum

Septal nuclei are situated in the forebrain and receive two main inputs; from the hippocampus via the fimbria and from the brainstem via the medial forebrain bundle. If the fimbria is cut, 30% of synapses in the septum degenerate

(Fig. 7–3a). The majority of the fibres from the hippocampus end on dendritic spines, and of these about 50% are removed (Fig. 7–3b). Since degeneration of the presynaptic terminal leaves the postsynaptic site vacant for a brief period, it may make contact with a glial element such as an astrocyte (Fig. 7–3c). Four weeks after the operation, the number of synapses has returned to normal. This is due to the production of new synapses, which may appear initially as double or multiple synapses (Fig. 7–3d). These subsequently give way to the conventional arrangement (Fig. 7–3e).

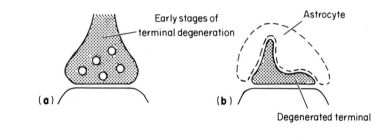

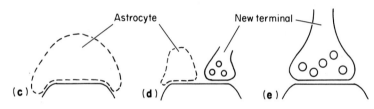

Fig. 7–3 Stages in the loss of degenerating synapses and production of new terminals in the septal region of the forebrain.

These new synapses probably result from sprouting of undamaged terminals from the medial forebrain bundle, which occupy synaptic sites vacated by degenerated hippocampal fibres. Whether such anomalous synapses are functional is not yet known.

7.3 Synaptic remodelling

Following degeneration, synapses may be re-formed in one of two ways. According to a *reoccupation model* postsynaptic sites are retained (Fig. 7–4a). Afferent fibres re-occupy sites vacated by degenerated terminals and proceed to form new synaptic junctions utilizing old postsynaptic sites. In spinal cord, new abnormal synapses have short synaptic contact regions, with a vacant postsynaptic site interspersed between them (Fig. 7–4a). According to this model, there is no change in synaptic numbers throughout the degeneration-regeneration cycle. An alternative model is a *de novo* one; postsynaptic sites are lost during

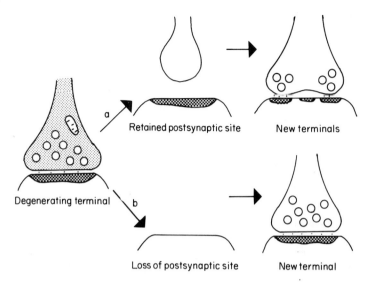

Fig. 7-4 Two models for synaptic remodelling following synaptic degeneration: (**a**) re-occupation model; (**b**) *de novo* formation.

degeneration and subsequently restored as synaptic sites are re-assembled (Fig. 7-4b).

Although the re-establishment of synaptic contacts is impressive, intermediate stages in synaptic maturation still need to be demonstrated. Unequivocal evidence regarding the extent to which new contact sites are established during reactive synaptogenesis is lacking, and one would like to have additional information about the nature of vacated postsynaptic specializations. It is even possible that reactive synaptogenesis prevents the re-establishment of normal synaptic connections; that could lead to a pathological situation.

7.4 Environment-induced plasticity

Neural plasticity underlies the brain's response to its environment. Evidence has been gradually increasing that psychotropic drugs, malnutrition, visual experience, hormonal levels, social isolation and events involved in learning, affect various facets of brain organization. These approaches have been supplemented by more subtle forms of environmental modification, involving alterations in the complexity of the sensory environment.

The development, morphology and functional state of the brain are dependent upon the nature of the environment in which the animal lives and on the level of stimulation to which it is subjected. Direct stimulation for as little as a few minutes produces morphological changes in visual and auditory tracts. In similar fashion, the learning of tasks brings about considerable structural and functional modification of the brain. More surprising, even very general differences in stimulation levels, such as those induced by rearing animals in environments of varying physical and social complexity, produce marked biochemical, physiological, endocrine, morphological and functional variations in brains.

The major environmental conditions employed are: *impoverished* (IC) in which a rat lives by itself in a small plain cage and remains relatively undisturbed; *social* (SC) with a few rats living together undisturbed in a larger cage; *enriched* (EC), much the same as SC, except that a selection of toys and objects is in the cage and is changed daily (Fig. 7–5).

Rats are generally placed in these cages at weaning (25 days old) and are left there for further periods up to 160 days. Maximum neural effects are obtained after 30 days of differential experience, although differences in brain structure have been reported after as little as four days. In switchover experiments rats are reared from weaning in either IC or EC environments, after which they are switched to the opposite environment for an equal period of time. An enriched environment in the second period (30 days) appears to overcome the effects of deprivation during the first period (30 days) and an enriched environment during the first 30 days affords some protection against effects of a subsequently impoverished environment. When longer periods of time are used, greater prolonged exposure to a secondary environment (enriched or impoverished) modifies and may even nullify the effects of the primary environment.

Data on which these ideas are based range from brain weight and length to the number and size of neurons and even to the number and size of synapses. In between these extremes the thickness of the cerebral cortex and the extent of dendritic branching have also been examined. Brains from rats living in enriched environments are heavier, have deeper cortices, larger neurons with longer and more complex branching dendrites, and larger but less numerous synapses. Protein and neurotransmitter changes occur in the brains of enriched rats.

Increases in dendritic complexity in EC rats are measured by an increase in the number of dendritic intersections, plus an increase in high-order branching (§ 2.2). The maximum dendritic response occurs in the occipital cortex, with enhanced branching patterns of pyramidal cell dendrites in the temporal and occipital cortices; no such enhancement has been described for equivalent neurons of the frontal cortex.

At the light microscope level information about the frequency of synaptic sites is provided by dendritic spines in Golgi-stained preparations. Using this criterion, EC rats have a higher frequency of synaptic sites than IC rats. This, coupled with the increased complexity of dendritic branching, points to an increase in the number of synapses per neuron in EC rats. Dendritic spines however, cannot be taken as a definitive guide to the presence of synapses.

Ultrastructural examination of synapses focuses attention on the absolute number of synapses per unit area or volume of tissue. No account is taken of the relationship between synaptic and neuronal numbers, nor between these parameters and the volume of the cortical region under investigation. Using ultrastructural parameters, EC rats have fewer, but longer, synapses than IC rats. These data are difficult to explain in terms of comparable light microscopical ones. An interesting additional parameter is that of sub-synaptic plate perforations; these are gaps in the postsynaptic thickening and are more frequent in larger synapses than small ones. The occipital cortex of EC rats has a significantly higher proportion of synapses with perforations than does that of IC rats.

Interesting as these findings are, it would be short-sighted to overlook how animals subjected to different environments actually behave. Of all tests of behavioural ability, maze-learning brings to the fore the consistently superior performance of the enriched animals. Certain other tests, such as discrimination-reversal learning, point in the same direction.

With both structural and behavioural results, effects vary. Some parts of the brain appear to be more susceptible to environmental variation than others, while animals react more at certain ages than others. The overall impression, however, is of a causal relationship between brain and environment.

7.5   Synaptic plasticity

The responses of synapses to malnutrition and barbiturate anaesthesia illustrate how labile synapses are and the value of using synaptic parameters as subtle indicators of neural plasticity. The maturity of synaptic junctions as structural units appears to be undermined by malnutrition. Throughout development in malnourished rat brains, there is a shift towards the immature end of the synaptic continuum. Presynaptic terminal parameters, such as vesicle number and packing, mitochondrial density, terminal area and synaptic length, are deficient up to 20 days postnatal in protein-deficient rat cerebral cortex. The curvature of synaptic junctions also shows marked differences in protein-deficient material, indicating perhaps a preponderance of inactive terminals compared with those from well-nourished material.

Barbiturates also modify synaptic curvature; in addition, they result in an increase in the number of vesicle-attachment sites (§ 5.4). With increasing doses of pentobarbitone there is a marked increase in curvature negativity (concave towards the presynaptic terminal), accompanied by an increase in synaptic length, dense projection numbers and terminal area. Reversal of the negativity trend at higher dose levels is paralleled by reversal of these accompanying trends. This, plus the increased frequency of vesicle attachment sites at the presynaptic membrane in unanaesthetized material, can be accounted for by recycling of membrane within the terminal.

Barbiturates exert an inhibitory effect on vesicular membrane transport and synaptic vesicle turnover. Their synaptic site of action can be detected and followed using ultrastructural techniques. This example of synaptic plasticity is reinforced by recent work, which has detected differences in unanaesthetized synaptic ultrastructure when different techniques for killing animals are employed. Moreover, barbiturates exert differential effects on synaptic ultra-structure at different ages throughout the developmental period.

Results of this nature show that minor variations in synaptic morphology can, not only be detected, but also assessed alongside functional considerations. It is hoped that, in time, synaptic organization and plasticity may throw light on the much broader issues of neuronal and even brain plasticity.

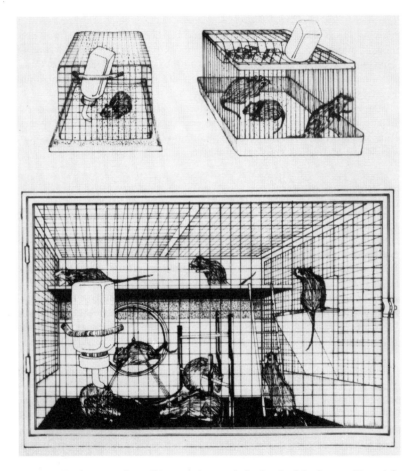

Fig. 7-5 Environmental conditions used to study brain plasticity in rats. Upper left, impoverished condition; upper right, social condition; lower, enriched condition.

Further Reading

BJÖRKLUND, A. and STENEVI, U. (1976). Regeneration of monoaminergic and cholinergic neurons in the mammalian central nervous system. *Physiological Reviews*, **59**, 62–100.

BULLOCK, T. H. (1977). *Introduction to Nervous Systems*. Freeman, San Francisco.

COTMAN, C. W. and LYNCH, G. S. (1976). Reactive synaptogenesis in the adult nervous system. In: *Neuronal Recognition*, S. H. Barondes (ed.). Plenum Press, New York.

COTTRELL, G. A. and USHERWOOD, P. N. R. (1977). *Synapses*. Blackie, Glasgow.

GREENOUGH, W. T. (1975). Experiential modification of the developing brain. *American Scientist*, **63**, 37–46.

HEUSER, J. E. (1977). Synaptic vesicle exocytosis revealed in quick-frozen frog neuro-muscular junctions treated with 4-aminopyridine and given a single electric shock. In: *Society for Neuroscience Symposia, Vol. 2*, W. M. Cowan and J. A. Ferrendelli (eds). Society for Neuroscience, Bethesda.

ISRAËL, M., DUNANT, Y. and MANARANCHE, R. (1979). The present status of the vesicular hypothesis. *Progress in Neurobiology*, **13**, 237–75.

JACOBSON, M. (1978). *Developmental Neurobiology*, 2nd edition. Plenum Press, New York.

JONES, D. G. (1975). *Synapses and Synaptosomes: Morphological Aspects*. Chapman and Hall, London.

JONES, D. G. (1981). Ultrastructural approaches to the organization of central synapses. *American Scientist*, **69**, 200–10.

KUFFLER, S. W. and NICHOLLS, J. G. (1976). *From Neuron to Brain*. Sinauer, Sunderland, Mass.

LUND, R. D. (1978). *Development and Plasticity of the Brain*. Oxford University Press, New York.

MESSENGER, J. B. (1979). *Nerves, Brains and Behaviour*. Studies in Biology no. 114. Edward Arnold, London.

PETERS, A., PALAY, S.L. and WEBSTER, H. de F. (1976). *The Fine Structure of the Nervous System*. Saunders, Philadelphia.

SHEPHERD, G. M. (1979). *The Synaptic Organization of the Brain*, 2nd edition. Oxford University Press, New York.

USHERWOOD, P. N. R. (1973). *Nervous Systems*. Studies in Biology no. 36. Edward Arnold, London.

ZIMMERMANN, H. (1979). Vesicle recycling and transmitter release. *Neuroscience*, **4**, 1773–804.

Subject Index